FINDING THE VOICE INSIDE YOU™

How I Lost Half of Myself,
Won Big,
and Am Living the Life
of My Dreams.

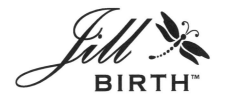

The future belongs to those
who believe in the beauty of their dreams.

– Eleanor Roosevelt

DEDICATION

First and foremost,
for my children Scott, Annie, and Zackery
who have taught me what is
most important in life

and

for my friends and family
who believed in me
even in those moments
when I had trouble
believing in myself.

CONTENTS

ACKNOWLEDGMENT

Thank you to my friend Carrie Curley;
without her, the dream
of writing this book
would never have
been realized.

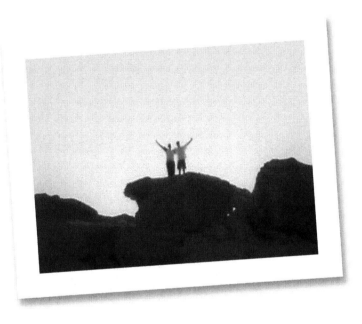

INTRODUCTION

I'm finally living my happily-ever-after life!
Now I work hard each and every day to pay it forward
and inspire others to make their dreams come true.

— Jill Birth

A couple of years ago I was visiting St. George, Utah. This gorgeous place was once the home of Mormon pioneers who grew cotton for a living. It is located near the Mojave Desert and the Pine Mountains. I was admiring one of those mountains when my oldest son, Scott, came up to me and said, "Hey Mom, let's go climb that mountain tomorrow morning."

My first response was to refuse. I had never climbed a mountain. And, in my mind, I was afraid I couldn't do it because I was too heavy. You see, I have been a professional dieter all my life, binging and dieting myself right up to 263 pounds. I'm an emotional eater, and when I fall, I fall big!

Beginning in 1998, determined to lose weight and get healthy once and for all, I would ask my husband or one of my friends to take my "before" pictures from the front, the side, and the back. I had 24 of those "before" pictures taken over the next several years. Although I had enough pictures to fill an entire scrapbook, you know what? There never was an "after" picture. I always allowed something to derail my resolve to get a handle on my food addiction.

I was no longer so morbidly obese on the day that Scott asked me to climb that mountain. By then, I had released about 80 pounds. Yet in my mind I was still that overweight woman who couldn't run or play with her kids. I had never hiked before, never mind climb a mountain. It took me a few minutes to conquer that shadowy inner self, then a warm feeling came over me and I felt as if someone whispered in my ear, "you can do it."

"Sure," I told Scott. "Let's climb that mountain together. It'll be fun."

We woke early the next morning, packed a lunch, and started our ascent. We didn't go as fast as Scott might have climbed with his friends, probably; however, I made it to the top easily. At the summit, we sat side-by-side, ate our lunches, and gazed out at the view.

Suddenly, Scott turned to me with tears in his eyes and said, "Thank you, Mom, for getting healthy for us."

I hugged him hard and vowed right then to never sit on the sidelines of life again. I was going to have enough confidence in myself to live my dreams, I decided, and I pledged to fulfill my goal of inspiring other people—people just like you—by showing you how to live a healthier life, too.

I know what it's like to struggle. Believe me, I know every excuse that people can give for not being able to lose weight and change their lives because I've probably used every one of those excuses myself. It's still a struggle for me some days not to revert to the old me and give in to my food addiction. There were some days that I literally made it through my weight loss and personal transformation on my knees, in prayer. Day by day, though, it became easier, as I felt myself changing inside and out.

If I can find the courage and strength to release weight and live a healthier life, you can, too. I'm going to show you how.

Releasing weight and getting healthy is an intimate journey, and it is unique for each of us. In the first part of this book, you'll read my personal story of pain and triumph, starting with my path to obesity and continuing through my struggles with motherhood and marriage. I know some parts of my story are painful. I'm choosing to share even these details because they demonstrate how sometimes we can only move forward in our lives by understanding the pain we've been through—and learning to let it go.

In the second part of the book, I'll help you map out your own success story. You'll learn simple, step-by-step strategies for putting your past behind you, dealing with your food addiction, and creating a vision for your future. You won't just release weight. You will discover how to live your dreams and take full advantage of the riches life has to offer as you find the courage to be the person you've always wanted to be. You'll learn how to accept, even embrace, the new you—for now and for ever. I'm going to help you find the voice within you, one step at a time.

By the time I completed my transformation, I had literally lost half of myself, going from 263 pounds to 132 pounds, and from a size 22 to a size 4. I could fit my hips and both legs into one leg of my old jeans. The process of meeting this challenge helped me gain the physical health and self-confidence to do many of the things I once only dreamed of doing—from running half-marathons to climbing mountains, from swimming to riding bikes with all three of my gorgeous kids.

This is my "happily ever after." Now I work every single day to pay it forward, hoping to inspire millions of people like you to find the same kind of confidence, drive, courage, and faith to become the person of *your* dreams.

I know that you can do it, because I will be walking beside you every step of the way.

JILL BIRTH

PART I: MY STORY

All your life there are going to be defining moments.
Turning points, where it will be up to you to decide
about something. And your job is always going to be
to know what is true for you, what's right,
and then act on it.

—Elizabeth Berg,
True to Form

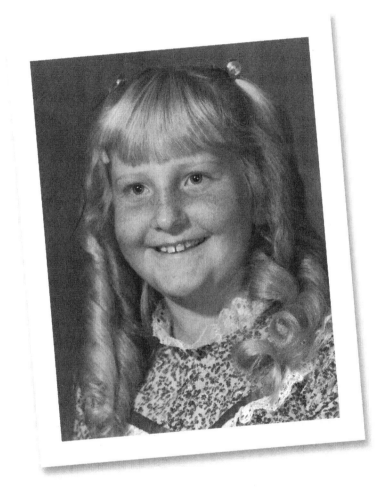

1

YOU ARE ONE FAT KID

People are my passion.

— Jill Birth

The first time I had to face the fact that I was overweight I was in third grade and only eight years old. The school nurse asked my classmates and me to stand in a line outside her office. One by one, she wanted each of us to step onto her scale so that she could measure our height and weight as part of our annual physical exams.

I already knew by then that I was bigger than everyone else—I had always been the tallest one in my class—so I went to the back of the line. I guess I hoped to avoid the whole ordeal somehow. Finally, though, it was my turn to step on that scale. When I did, I weighed 142 pounds.

The nurse stared at me in horror. "Oh my heck, you are one fat little kid!" she cried. "You weigh more than me, and I'm 20 years older than you are. You need to go home and have your mom put you on a diet!"

Naturally, the minute I got home, I started bawling my head off. "The school nurse says I'm too fat and need to be on a diet!" I told my mother.

I'm sure it must have broken my mother's heart to see me so upset. She had been struggling with weight issues all her life—not just with her own but, with my two sisters' as well. My mom was always on some kind of diet, trying to lose about 20 pounds of extra weight. My oldest sister, Lesa, was also overweight.

To complicate matters in our family, my other sister, Laurel, was anorexic—to the point where, in junior high, my parents worried that they might have to hospitalize her. Consequently, my mother was always trying to get Laurel to gain weight by feeding her fattening foods and ice cream, while at the same time keeping herself, Lesa, and me on a strict diet to help slim us down. It couldn't have been easy for her.

It wasn't easy for me, either. After that nurse's heartless comment, my mother whisked me straight off to a Weight Watchers meeting the next day. Although the group was supportive, I was still such a young kid that I found it tough to resist the tasty foods other children my age loved to eat, like pizza or macaroni and cheese.

When I look back on my early childhood, it's clear that I was an emotional eater; however, it's tough to pinpoint when or why I first became truly addicted to food. I had a pleasant childhood. My parents were happily married. There was never any physical, emotional, or sexual abuse in my family. We all got along and loved each other.

My family is devout in our faith—we belong to the Church of Jesus Christ of Latter-Day Saints (LDS). In the LDS church, a ward is the larger of two types of local congregations (the smaller one is called a branch). A ward is presided over by a bishop, the equivalent of a pastor in many other Christian religions. My father was a bishop for the ward in which we were members. Each ward can have anywhere from 200 to 500 people in it within a reasonable travel time of the meetinghouse, and, because my dad was a bishop, we kids were expected to be stellar examples for the children in the rest of the ward.

It was hard sometimes because whenever I did something wrong, I would feel so guilty, particularly if it was something that I knew might earn my parents' disapproval. At the same time, I always felt secure in the knowledge that our parents loved us.

The dominant personality in our family for sure was my mom: a noisy, fun-loving woman who could still go crazy having fun even as an adult. She has always been a joyful kid-at-heart. For instance, Mom is the one who taught me just how much fun it can be to toilet paper a house. Whenever she wanted to have a little fun with somebody, she'd get together with me and a big group of my friends and we'd head over to the grocery store, stock up on toilet paper, and sneak out at night to weave it through the trees and bushes around the houses of relatives, friends, my sister's boyfriends—just about anybody was fair game.

I remember, too, shortly after I got my learner's permit, Mom, one of my friends, and I were driving down Main Street in our car when she said, "Get in the driver's seat, Jill, and I'll hide in the back seat."

"But I don't have my license," I protested. "Oh, come on!" she urged. "Do it! It'll be fun!" I did, and, yes, it was fun. With my mom's encouragement, I felt daring and brave!

Everyone in town knew my mother for her great sense of humor and fun ways. My mom was so much fun that most of my friends loved her more than they loved me, for sure. She was easy to talk to and just had this way of being supportive and being a friend to everyone.

My dad was much quieter than my mother and didn't like to cause a fuss about anything. Whenever we would do something silly, we would come in telling my dad all about it. He would shake his head, smile with a sheepish grin, and peer at us with a sort of an "Oh no, what are they up to now?" look on his face. It makes me smile when I think about it to this day.

I'm fun like my mom, yet I dislike confrontations just like my dad. I guess you could say that I'm a people pleaser: I've always been the sort of person who loves other people; I don't like to disappoint anyone; if there is ever anyone in need, I will do whatever I can to help.

With a happy marriage, six kids, and only one modest schoolteacher's salary, our family had a lot of love, yet not a whole lot of money to go around. We wore hand-me-down clothes and lived in a modest brick rambler on a couple of acres of land in Pleasant View, Utah. My grandparents, aunts, and uncles lived close by and it was beautiful and peaceful up on our mountain. The town was small and most of the families were LDS. There wasn't even a town center, really, or a single stoplight. I still remember how much fun it was to sled down the snowy main streets of town in the winter.

In addition to Dad's salary as a teacher, we owned a 50-acre cherry orchard a few minutes' drive from our home that we relied on for additional income. Some of my favorite childhood memories include picking fruit with my family. We would pick from the cherry orchard as well as from the pear and peach trees on my parents' property. We're talking a massive production here, like 27 bushels of pears and 500 quarts of peaches a year in addition to all of those cherries!

My entire extended family pitched in at harvest time, so we all knew the meaning of hard work from an early age. We hired a ton of kids from around town to help out, too. It's an exciting kind of work because most of the cherry harvesting is done at night. We'd all go out to the orchard at about 10 o'clock in the evening. Machines clamp onto the trees to shake cherries onto nets. The cherries are then dumped into a trailer filled with water; the water is cold and keeps the cherries cool and fresh until they're transported in bins to the factory where they're canned and sent off to various distributors. The best part? Because we picked the cherries at night, we frequently had sleepovers in our house and kids hung around our house all summer long.

Sounds like an idyllic childhood, right? Yet, looking back, I remember being obsessed with food and feeling hungry all of the time. I know now that, by first grade, I was truly addicted to food. I remember sitting in the school cafeteria during lunch and wanting to eat all of the food on my friends' trays; one day, I had four hamburgers on my tray and ate them all. Whatever my friends didn't want to eat I totally ate, and that remained true right through elementary school.

Having my mom take me to Weight Watchers just made things worse, I think, because I rebelled against the idea that I could only have two boiled eggs and half a cup of cottage cheese or something like that for a meal. Even then, I had an "all or nothing" kind of personality; if you tell me I can't have something, I want it all the more! I even began hoarding food in my bedroom—taking the sweet, fattening stuff my mother bought for my skinny sister, Laurel, and hiding it to eat later.

Some people blame the media for how women become overly self-conscious about our bodies and begin to link our self-esteem and confidence to how we look on the outside. I don't think that was true in my case. While I do worry about that now with my own daughter, my family didn't even own a television until I was 12 years old. Even if there was something in the media, my mother and sisters never discussed body image in that way.

So how did I first start feeling self-conscious about my size? In addition to that nurse in third grade being so tactless and outspoken about my weight, other people in my life made me the object of criticism or even ridicule. At school, for instance, the main message was the same as it is today: skinny kids are cool and fat kids are not. A lot of my classmates made fun of me because I couldn't do the kinds of things in gym class that the other kids could do, like run laps around the gym. It didn't help that I had a large nose—that was just one more reason for hurtful comments. Family members also added to my feeling of hurt. Even my own uncle would pinch my roll of belly fat occasionally and say, "If you can pinch an inch, you're too fat!"

Meanwhile, at home it was abundantly clear that being thin meant successfully attracting boys to date and—in the LDS tradition— to marry in the temple. In the LDS faith, we're asked not to date until we're 16 and to remain chaste until after marriage. When my heavy sister, Lesa, went off to college, my mom worried less about Lesa and boyfriends, and more about her health. She'd say things like, "I wonder how Lesa's doing with her weight, eating all of that college food."

On the other hand, my mother lived vicariously through my sister Laurel, who I saw as "the chosen one" because she was the one who got all of the attention from boys. Actually, we all lived vicariously through Laurel, I think, by peeking our heads out to watch her on the door step with her dates.

"I wonder if she's going to kiss him tonight," Mom would muse, and I would envy what seemed like my sister Laurel's perfect life. When I grew up, I fantasized that I might have a figure just like her.

*

Despite being heavy in elementary school, I was an active child. That's probably the reason I was overweight though not yet morbidly obese. Soccer was my best sport. I played defense on an all-star soccer team; I was so strong that I once scored a goal while making a kickoff from center field.

This glorious athletic career was cut short in sixth grade, though, when I broke my ankle playing soccer. I really started piling on the pounds in junior high because I wasn't nearly as active as I had been before. My mother was still keeping me on a Weight Watchers sort of diet at home, yet whenever I went to friends' houses, I knew I wasn't going to stick to boiled eggs and chicken. I'd have candy or pizza, and I still did a lot of closet eating. Whatever we had in our house that I wasn't supposed to eat, I made sure to hide it so that I could eat it in secret. The result of doing this was that I felt terrible. I knew it was dishonest, and no matter how much I thought I wanted the food at the time, eating it made me feel awful about myself afterward, both physically and emotionally.

I'm grateful that the Lord made up for my body challenges by blessing me with a cheerful, outgoing, people-loving personality. Have you ever noticed that some overweight people seem like they're the happiest people on Earth? That was me. I really love everyone, regardless of what path they are taking through life.

I have the gift of a loving heart from God, and I might not have realized that gift if I hadn't had to struggle so hard to manage my weight. I think that, when you're overweight, you often learn to compensate for what you don't like about yourself physically by becoming friendlier than everyone else around you, hoping to fit in. Who can dislike a smiling person who always has nice things to say, right?

That was my best defense, and I used it wisely. As a result, I had tons of friends throughout junior high and high school. In fact, by high school I actually took the student directory and studied it, checking off the names of everyone I didn't know and making it a point to become friends with those people. I wanted everyone to have a friend, even if it was only me, and I made a point of saying "hi" to everyone I met.

I was a solid B student and popular enough to be elected into student government. I mainly worked behind the scenes because I was too insecure to stand up and speak in front of people—something I do now with ease. I still remember the agony of having to do a presentation in English class and bursting into tears because I just couldn't get up there and speak in front of my classmates. I was too self-conscious about my weight to be a confident public speaker. Standing in front of people, they could look at me head on and couldn't help but see how heavy I was.

Throughout high school, when summer rolled around, I'd vow to lose 20 or 30 pounds and start the next school year off thinner (and more popular with boys, I hoped). I'd start out being really good—exercising and eating right. It was tough because every summer that would be my biggest goal. I was always optimistic at first, then when the weight wouldn't come off as quickly as I'd liked it to, I would start believing in the back of my mind that I'd probably fail just like the summer before.

Between my sophomore and junior years of high school, I finally had my nose fixed. That boosted my confidence a little. Yet, it was still tough to always feel so left out or even shunned by a lot of the other kids. The teachers weren't much better. I remember one gym teacher who was ornery all the time. She would single me out and yell at me whenever I couldn't do the laps around the football field with my class. "Hurry up! Run faster!" that teacher would scream at me. It was so humiliating that I'd want to cry. I tried to keep up with the other kids, but I just couldn't do it.

I was hurt, too, because even though some of my good friends were boys, I was never, ever asked to a school dance by any of them. Instead, they would befriend me just to get to know my friends in the hope of dating them. I was a mother figure and matchmaker to just about everyone, and watched my friends go to prom, boys' choice dances, and the homecoming dance while I stayed home.

The girls' dramas were sometimes even worse than having boys ignore me. I had one really good friend in junior high who just dropped me completely when we got to high school because she found cooler, thinner friends, and that really hurt. Even now, when I think about how mean and condescending some of those girls were, I can remember so clearly how horrible they made me feel.

My mom called me a "social butterfly" because I had so many activities after school. But deep down, I knew that I didn't really have any true friends other than my cousin Kristen. I often went home and cried at night because the girls I went to school with could be so phony and unkind.

*

How big was I? The truth is that I was overweight, yet not hugely obese by today's standards. I was tall—about 5' 9" by the start of high school—and I probably weighed about 170 pounds. I was about a size 14, though, and that was much, much bigger than most of the teeny little girls in my high school.

So, as I said, every summer I tried to lose weight. And every summer, I'd lose some pounds—then put them right back on. In addition to Weight Watchers, I probably tried every other weight loss plan there was, including the ones where you'd buy their food and bring it home. I'd do well when I stayed on the diet, then, of course, I'd go off the diet and bounce right back up the scale.

Plus, the weight loss was slow. At the Weight Watchers meetings, the other members would cheer if you lost a pound a week. The problem was that I had so much to lose that I got frustrated, thinking, "What? I just starved myself all week and lost only one pound? Are you kidding me?" I understood that the members were trying to be supportive of one another, but I just couldn't get excited about losing weight a pound at a time—not when I had so many extra pounds! Instead, I felt overwhelmed and discouraged.

The whole process of losing weight became so overwhelming that

I would just quit. I'd think, "Oh my goodness, how am I going to lose 30 pounds in just three months over the summer?" I'd be depressed enough to quit whatever diet I was on before I even really gave it a try because I was so sure it wouldn't work and lacked the self-confidence to continue trying.

At the same time, the fact that I couldn't lose weight altered how I lived. I don't think I realized how much at the time, but I do now. After hot nights and days of harvesting cherries for hours at a time, for example, my whole family and all of our friends who'd been working so hard together would reward themselves by traveling to a water slide park, about 20 minutes away, to have fun and cool off.

But guess what? I never wanted to join in the fun. I knew that, if I climbed up those steps in a bathing suit, I would feel ashamed. People would be rolling their eyes and making snide, hurtful comments about my body behind my back. I would end up going anyway because I felt as though I would draw more attention to myself if I didn't, yet, all the while I felt humiliated by putting myself out there.

My whole life revolved around my weight. If I got up and weighed myself in the morning, I was on top of the world if my weight was down a little, yet I felt like a beast if I was up a few pounds. Despite my seemingly idyllic family life, supportive parents, and activities in high school, the real me was trapped somewhere deep inside myself. It wasn't a happy place to be.

Maybe that's why I married as young as I did—to leave all of that unhappiness behind and escape into a new life.

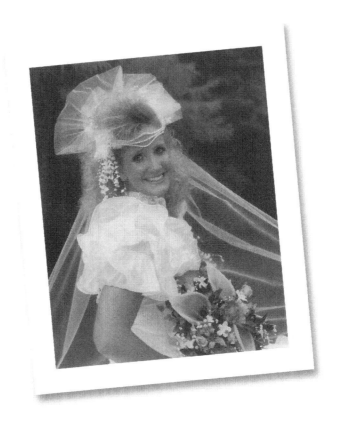

2

THE UNHAPPY PRINCESS BRIDE

Where would we be without goals?
Drifting, and probably not even doing *that* very well.

— Jill Birth

I 've always worked hard. In addition to helping my mom out around the house and pitching in to pick and can fruits and vegetables for our personal use, I held down jobs outside the house from the time I was 14 years old. My very first job was in a pizza shop, of all places. I loved it because I worked with a lot of fun people, yet, naturally, this wasn't the best kind of place for a pizza-loving food addict like me to work. You can imagine how that job helped me pack on the pounds!

In high school, one of my older brothers was the manager of a frozen yogurt place, and he hired me. I swirled frozen yogurt through my sophomore and junior years of high school. Because it was near the college, a lot of college kids frequented the place and a few of the guys began paying attention to me. This—plus not scarfing down pizza quite so often—led me to shed some weight. As I lost a few pounds and met more people, it dawned on me that some day I, too, would be in college and could maybe meet cute guys like these.

Something clicked in my mind, and there was my motivation! I began to really commit to losing weight. In addition to eating a little less, I had started playing soccer again by high school. I also mapped out a loop and started walking five miles a day, which led to an all-time low weight of 140 pounds—a fairly trim weight for a woman who is 5' 9" tall and somewhat athletic. I started feeling pretty good about myself at last.

My sister, Laurel, meanwhile, had started working in a local dentist's office as a dental assistant, and when one of the other assistants went on maternity leave, she got me a part-time position there. This proved to be the career I had been looking for without even knowing it! I started with small jobs, like filing and answering phones, and gradually took on more responsibilities. I was a hard worker and a reliable employee, so the dentists rewarded me by showing me the ropes and teaching me how to be a good dental assistant, which I'm so grateful for to this day.

My sister was a dental assistant, and my brother is an oral surgeon. So, needless to say, I had a lot of encouragement from my family to pursue a career in this field. Even without that family support, though, I would have loved it. I know a lot of people probably will think this is weird, but I'm a real tooth freak. I've loved teeth since I was just a little girl. As a child, before I went to bed, I'd go over each of my teeth with a toothpick. Crazy, huh? It's true!

Now, for the first time in my life, I could see my future unfolding: I would earn my college degree, pursue a career as a dental hygienist, fall in love, then marry the man of my dreams and have children. My life definitely didn't turn out quite the way I planned.

*

As I graduated from high school with my new, leaner body,

I continued with my resolve to stay fit and keep the weight off. No matter what the weather, I would walk that five-mile loop I had mapped out. Because I had to pay for my own college education, I continued working and living at home once I started college classes. Even so, I was thrilled to be in the exciting new social environment that college offered, one where no one had any idea what I used to look like or the struggles I'd had with my weight. It was a fresh start.

Back in those days, you didn't register online for classes. You had to stand in line at the registrar's office. This led to some interesting class selections on my part, because I'd see a cute guy in line in front of me, listen to him talk with his friends about whatever classes he was taking, and sign up for the same ones. We would start talking in class and I would sometimes get asked out on a date! It certainly wasn't like high school.

With my trim size and long, blonde hair, you can bet that I earned a lot of attention from guys. People who had known me in high school would stop me on campus and say, "Wow, Jill, you look so good!" It was wonderful and very different from what I was used to.

No, I still wasn't nearly as tiny as some of the really cute, pretty, college girls, yet I got enough attention to boost my ego a bit and make me feel more confident about myself. I was having the time of my life. Meanwhile, I started taking the core classes I'd need to study in the state college's dental hygiene program—lots of biology and chemistry classes that really challenged me academically. It was so much harder than high school.

Sometimes my college friends and I traveled down to Salt Lake City to a place that offered country swing dancing—something I could now enjoy doing because I wasn't nearly as self-conscious about my body. It was on one of these trips, in December of my freshman year, that I met Dave, my husband-to-be. He was a young man from a good LDS family, had recently returned from completing his mission, and was in school studying to become a mechanic.

Now, in the LDS culture, it's common to marry a returned missionary. LDS missionaries serve all over the world as volunteer representatives of the faith, not only proselyting, but also performing humanitarian aid work and serving in church-related activities.

I think I was even more attracted to Dave because, even though he had these apparent "good boy" qualities, I was attracted to wild boys, and that he was. Now, here was a scruffy, attractive, wild-looking guy—over six feet tall, with dark eyes and a handsome face—who came from a great family and was a returned missionary. He was the complete fantasy package. I was thrilled to meet him and to feel that zing of physical attraction between us.

After meeting and talking to him that first weekend, I started dating Dave steadily—so steadily that, when I had a trip planned with some friends to West Yellowstone for a snowmobiling weekend, Dave didn't want me to go. I went anyway and had a blast. Maybe that's why Dave was in such a hurry to propose to me; we were engaged by Valentine's Day. And, because Dave said he wouldn't wait for me if I served my mission first, I said yes. Now I could finally start my married life!

Remember that I'd suffered through many years of not being at all attractive to boys, years of eating in secret and feeling lonely and lost. How could I possibly imagine a better future than this one? I couldn't. Little did I know how far from my fantasy this future would turn out to be.

*

Dave and I were married in the LDS temple and we invited over 800 well-wishers to the reception. I felt like the "Princess of the Day" in my ruffled dress with puff sleeves, despite the killer 90-degree heat flattening everyone's hair and causing perspiration to pour down our faces.

For people who practice the LDS faith, marriage means making a sacred covenant with the Lord. Your marriage is for eternity. These are serious vows and I made them with all my heart, despite being just barely 20 years old and only having known this man for a few short months.

All of my life, I had dreamed of someday falling in love and having a fairy tale wedding with the blessing of friends and family. Now that my special day was here, I could only hope that I might quickly learn how to be a good wife and make my husband happy.

Our marriage didn't start out as the fairy tale I had imagined. I learned that although you love someone, it doesn't necessarily mean that you know them. The first days of our marriage were overwhelming. I felt as though I may have been a little too innocent to be married just yet. Although the honeymoon started out a bit rocky, I just prayed that our love for one another would make up for what little we knew of each other.

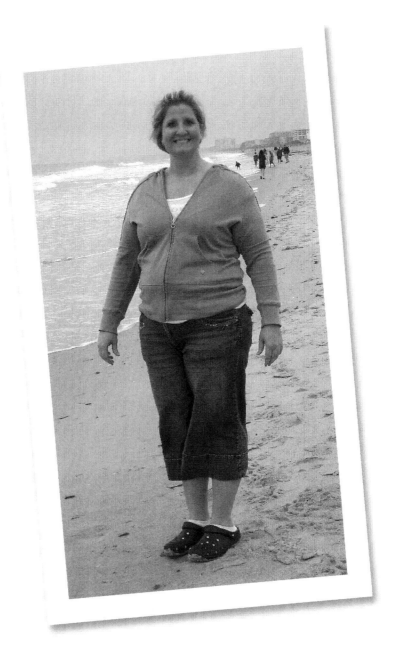

3

MARRIAGE, MOTHERHOOD, AND MISERY

Our greatest glory is not in never failing, but in rising up every time we fail.

— Ralph Waldo Emerson

After the honeymoon, Dave and I moved into an apartment in a duplex in Ogden, about 10 minutes away from my parents' house. It soon became clear that our marriage had gotten off on the wrong foot. Or, to put it another way, we were out of sync as husband and wife. I felt like we were destined to keep stepping on each other's toes. I wasn't sure if we would ever learn to understand each other.

For instance, during our honeymoon, I wanted to call my mom just to check in; I was used to doing that kind of thing and saw no reason to stop. I just wanted to tell her that we had arrived safely because I knew she'd be worried. Dave made fun of me for this. He seemed jealous and annoyed that I still wanted to be close to my mother after our marriage.

I was angry at him for making fun of me and wanted, if only briefly, to run home to my mom. And I was sad, too, because I could see that Dave was already trying to control who I could talk to and visit with so early in our marriage. When we returned to Utah, Dave announced that he didn't want my mother visiting our apartment. "I don't want her meddling in our business," he explained. I was heartbroken.

Now that I'm older and so many years have gone by, I can see why he felt that way. Dave wasn't much older than I was—hardly past his teen years—so I'm sure that he was working hard to figure out what it meant to be an independent adult and a good husband, just as I was struggling to define my career and be a good wife. He didn't feel that I should need my mom now that I was married to him, I guess. However, at the time, I found this wish of his to be a difficult one to honor. My mom and I have always been extremely close, partly because I was the baby of the family by many years and partly because I had always lived at home.

My friends began noticing that I had changed since my marriage. Before, I had always been ready to smile and laugh at just about anything. But, now I was becoming subdued and more introverted.

To add to my stress, Dave and I were struggling financially. He decided to focus on working as a welder instead of finishing his college degree, while at the same time resenting me because I had convinced him that we should live near my job in the dental office rather than find a place close to his family and school in Salt Lake City.

Dave earned a decent hourly wage, yet not enough that I could quit my job at the dentist's office. He tried to supplement his income by guiding people on hunting trips, sometimes for weeks at a time. For my part, I also tried to add to our household revenue stream by performing extra jobs—anything from selling candles to doing yard work for other people.

Our worries about money and our long work days did nothing for our post-honeymoon marital state. Dave was doing his best to be a good provider and husband and I was trying to be a good wife to him in return. Yet, nothing we did seemed to be enough for us to stay connected emotionally—or to get us ahead financially.

It seemed that Dave also had some trust issues. If I came home later than expected, he would grill me on where I had been. Dave's need to know my every move led me to sometimes lie about my whereabouts just to evade the third degree. Dave would show his disappointment if he didn't like my answers. Again, this was partly because of his inability to feel comfortable with my parents. He seemed to avoid them whenever possible.

I take full responsibility for not being straightforward with Dave at times. I just wanted to be able to see my family without arguing about it with him every time I visited them.

I think that part of the issue Dave had with my parents is that my mom definitely wears the pants in our family. She is an assertive woman and Dave was probably afraid that I'd turn out just like her and try to boss him around if I continued to spend time with her, even though I'm more apt to avoid confrontations, like my dad.

In addition to wanting to control my relationships, Dave tried to control my looks. When I talked about cutting my hair, he said that it was grounds for divorce because he wanted a wife with long, blonde hair. On more than one occasion, he even went so far as to measure my hair before a haircut and again afterward, just to make sure that it was the length he wanted and not one-half-inch less. Once, I cut it all off in a fit of fury just to call his bluff because I was so sick of this power struggle between us. It was a small attempt at having some sort of control. I know it seems silly. Would he really leave me if I cut my hair?

In truth, I was so inexperienced at being in relationships that I often didn't know what to do when we disagreed and tended to shut down. I just knew that I was unhappy. I tried to be more understanding about how different Dave and I were and struggled to view his desire to know my every move as a sign that he really loved me and treasured our marriage. I hoped that these sorts of adjustments were typical of every newly married couple's struggle to learn how to live together.

The unfortunate result of our rocky relationship, however, was that every time Dave disagreed with me about something, I took his remarks as criticism and began to believe that I wasn't good enough or pretty enough to be his wife. My early attempts to lose weight through yo-yo dieting represented my efforts to please him—and to have at least one area of my life where I felt like I had some control.

*

Speaking of yo-yo dieting, it was common for me during those early years of our marriage to lose 20 pounds on some drastic diet—like eating only grapefruit or cabbage soup—and then gain those pounds right back again, plus a few more. This time in my life was an emotional roller coaster ride as well as a physical one, not just for me, but for Dave, too. At that point I had lost hope of releasing the weight and keeping off. I was able to hide it behind a smile on my face with everyone other than my husband. Poor Dave must have felt like he was living with a beast.

Because Dave's mother was a large woman, and because I had been honest with Dave about my struggles with weight in the past, I honestly never imagined that my weight might become an issue in our marriage. I wholeheartedly believed—and still do—that being married means taking the bad with the good and working as a team. To me, marriage means vowing to love your spouse inside even more than you love how he or she looks on the outside.

Dave felt differently, apparently. Or perhaps he didn't really know how he, himself, felt about my rapid ups and downs on the scale. I can't blame him for that. I would imagine it's tough for any spouse to marry someone who looks a certain way, only to discover that this partner is going to look completely different a short time later.

In any case, Dave sent me mixed messages. If I gained weight, my husband would sometimes point out a movie star with a great body and say, "If you could only look like her!" He probably thought that he was motivating me to control my weight; however, these sorts of remarks just broke my heart.

Other times, though, Dave was extremely supportive. When I'd start a new diet, he might say, "I believe in you, Jill. You can do this!" He would cheer me on over every lost ounce.

Once I was thin, though, he made his true feelings known, saying things like, "I hope you don't ever go back to being fat again. You just weren't attractive to me." When he said things like that, it honestly made me want to eat a Snickers bar! Dave also made comments about other overweight women, like, "I don't dig fat chicks." Or, if Dave saw a large woman taking a stroll, he might say, "Keep on walking. You need to burn off the fat," not realizing that I was internalizing all of this.

Just as I had chopped off my hair to see if Dave would love me without it, subconsciously, at least, my weight became a control issue between us. When I look back on that time now, I understand that I blamed Dave's critical remarks for making me feel bad about myself, when, in fact, self-esteem and confidence have to come from within. Nobody else can make you feel confident other than you—nor should anyone else have that responsibility, not even your spouse! It is up to you to find your own path to happiness and contentment.

Of course, I wasn't cognizant of any of that back then the way I am now. I had no idea that I was probably putting weight on just to test whether Dave would really stay with me if I were hugely obese, proving, "See, he loves me."

Oddly, whenever I did start gaining weight and went into the inevitable tailspin of despair, Dave was just as likely to comfort me as criticize me. He'd often say, "If you're going to be heavy, then just be happy the way you are." It was both confusing and unsettling to hear Dave's opinions about my weight, because I never knew what to expect.

Dave's mixed emotions about having a large wife—or a thin one—probably tapped right back into his childhood, which is when most of us form our impressions of what size is "best" or even "normal." His father, for instance, loved large women. Whenever I was at a heavy weight, Dave's dad was apt to tell me how beautiful I was. "I'm so glad you're a Cadillac," my father-in-law would say. "I don't like those little Beetle bugs." If I lost weight, though, Dave's dad would say, "Oh, you don't look as good now," and shake his head disapprovingly. "I liked you the way you were before."

Just as it wasn't easy for me to understand or control my

weight gains and losses, I'm sure it couldn't have been easy for Dave to live with a wife whose whole identity was wrapped up in her size and shape, as mine was. My moods could swing rapidly up or rapidly down depending on that number I saw on the scale every morning. I let my weight determine how happy I was. In fact, at one point, things were so bad that Dave wrote on the bathroom scale in permanent marker. The message was clear: "I am evil. Do not use!"

Sometimes I wondered if he could be right. Yet I couldn't disentangle my emotions from my food addiction, or my self-confidence from my weight, no matter how hard I tried. And oh, how I tried! I just wasn't ready to understand why I kept failing.

*

I was taking birth control pills when we were first married, yet I got pregnant within three months of our honeymoon. I felt sick and exhausted almost all of the time, but I didn't care. I was excited about my impending motherhood. I had been raised to believe that marrying and having children should be among your top goals in life, especially if you're a woman. I was also somehow convinced that having a baby would bring Dave and me closer. Boy, was I wrong!

Being pregnant allowed me to give up again on losing weight, because it gave me an excuse to eat for two, and I used that excuse, believe me! I knew that I wanted a healthy baby; I decided that I would focus on eating healthy foods and not worry about my weight again until after I was holding my baby in my arms. I simply let go of any attempts to control how much I ate, using my pregnancy as a handy reason for why I needed seconds at almost every meal and ice cream or pie for dessert—or even for breakfast! I would go so far as to tell Dave that I was heading to the gym to work out, when in reality I would go to the ice cream shop and sit on the lawn there to gorge on ice cream.

Doing this had disastrous results. Before my pregnancy was over, I had gained a whopping 80 pounds. I was no longer a pleasingly curvy woman. I was now officially obese by anyone's standards, tipping the scale at 225 pounds. Little did I know that this wasn't the heaviest I'd ever be.

While the birth of my first son, Scott, brought feelings of joy and tenderness more powerful than any other emotions I'd felt in my life, adjusting to motherhood was much more of a challenge than I had dreamed possible. In addition to being completely sleep-deprived and overwhelmed as any new mother is while learning how to care for her first child, I faced a huge hurdle when I tried to breastfeed my baby. The truth is that nursing just didn't work for me. It proved to be so difficult that I was concerned about Scott's nutrition and finally had to give up and feed my baby boy formula.

This failure caused a significant rift with Dave's family, because they equated breastfeeding with being a good mom. Whenever Scott became ill after that—at one point, he had to have his tonsils out because he had so many sore throats—Dave's family actually said to me that they believed Scott was sickly because I didn't breastfeed. How could I be such a failure after having this beautiful baby boy?

I was so vulnerable as a person, and so frightened at times by the responsibilities of new motherhood, that I started to believe that I really was a failure as a mom. Yet, at the same time, I knew differently in my heart. Scott had a sweet, peaceful personality, and he was my little buddy. We did everything together. And, because Dave was gone so often, my son and I formed a tight bond during those first few years. I learned that breastfeeding didn't make you a good mom. Showing your child love did.

At this point in my life, I hadn't yet realized that I was addicted to food or understood that I was an emotional eater. I ate when I was unhappy to comfort myself, and I ate when I was nervous. I ate when I wanted to reward myself for a job well done, and I ate when I felt angry and powerless, as I did much of the time in my marriage.

Food was my best friend. It was also taking charge of my life. All I could think about was what I was going to eat next. I didn't eat to survive. I lived to eat. The results were disastrous for my self-esteem, my health, and, ultimately, my marriage. I blamed my unhappiness on my weight, yet I think I was just unhappy in every area of my life. My weight was a reflection of my unhappiness. I hadn't yet connected the dots between my weight fluctuations and my deep-seated emotions.

*

From our apartment in Ogden, we moved in with Dave's brother and his wife in Centerville while we saved money to build a house in Clinton, about half an hour away. I loved living with Dave's brother and sister-in-law, who also struggled with her weight. She and I exercised a lot together and pushed each other to stay motivated and lose weight.

Again, as before the pregnancy, I tried every diet plan under the sun, even a strictly hot dog and bologna diet! Seriously! If one of my patients or one of the girls I worked with came into the office claiming that she'd found a diet that would guarantee losing seven pounds in seven days, all of the girls in our office would go right on it, in a frenzy, to try and lose weight, often with me leading the charge.

I lost weight, then gained it again, probably because I'd often reward myself for that initial 10-pound weight loss with a huge dinner and a couple of desserts because I'd been so "good." I had one patient in the dental office—another big lady—who would come in for her appointment and say, "So, what diet are you trying now?"

We would talk about our diets, and she would laugh when she said, "Well, looks like that diet's not working for you." I would laugh along with her while feeling horrible inside. Did she realize how humiliating that comment was?

She was right, though. Nothing I did to lose weight worked until I tried fen-phen. Fen-phen is a combination of fenfluramine or dexfenfluramine and phentermine. This drug, once widely used in the U.S., is no longer readily available due to the large amounts of fraud and the manufacture of counterfeit pills and to the abuse of this drug by some. Also, fen-phen could have serious side effects, including heart issues, blurred vision, irritability, sleeplessness, upset stomach, changes in sex drive, and dry mouth.

I loved it, however, as did many of the girls who worked in my office as well as my sister-in-law. Taking fen-phen allowed me to lose the weight and keep it off. The drug gave me a ton of energy also. A friend of mine who worked in a doctor's office prescribed the pills for me because she had seen her patients release weight so successfully while taking them. On fen-phen—which feels a lot like taking speed—I could clean the house in no time at all and I had the energy to work out every day. It seemed perfect.

Not that I needed to exercise to keep the pounds off! Thanks to fen-phen, my new best friend, I could eat only pizza and still stay thin. My appetite was so diminished that a single piece of pizza was now enough to keep me going all day and all night, too.

I didn't mind that I had trouble sleeping on fen-phen, because I had so much more energy and felt good about the way I looked. Dave finally seemed happy with the way I looked and I was actually noticed by other men as well, even if I just happened to be walking into a store or down the street. I felt comfortable with my appearance for the first time in my adult life.

With the help of fen-phen, I managed to whittle off all of my postpartum weight and more. I had finally achieved a figure that pleased my husband, yet I wasn't much happier. Frankly, it ticked me off that people treated me so differently just because I was thin. I didn't understand why. My heart was the same. I was more confused than ever about my own self-worth and where it really came from.

Once fen-phen became impossible to get, however, the weight crept back onto my body. I hadn't learned any good eating habits. I just took a pill that suppressed my appetite and hyped me up so much I couldn't sit still. Around that time, Dave and I decided to have another child. It wasn't long before my marriage was once again tense instead of the happily-ever-after I had dreamed about as a little girl.

*

Why, when our relationship was still so precarious, did I want another child? The answer was the same as always: I hoped it would bring my husband and me closer. However getting pregnant this time proved to be an ordeal. Being on fen-phen had affected my body in such a way that I had only sporadic periods. This disruption in my menstrual cycle caused us to have trouble conceiving; by the time Scott was three years old, I was taking fertility drugs which only made me gain more weight.

I tried to convince myself that I didn't care. It proved to be true once again that, if I was heavier, Dave was less interested in me. Although I didn't really understand this until later, my weight still posed a welcomed barrier between us.

Dave was making pretty good money now as a welder and I was still at the dental office. My mom as well as a good friend took care of Scott, who wasn't yet in preschool, so that I could keep working. We had enough income to qualify for a loan to build a house in a brand-new subdivision a patient had told me about. We hadn't saved any money, however, that didn't matter. We were first-time homebuyers and the banks didn't require much of a down payment for young couples like us back then.

In my mind, buying a house seemed like a smart investment, especially because the money we'd spend each month on the mortgage wasn't much more than the monthly rent we'd been paying for our apartment in Ogden. I knew that we could handle the payments on what we were making and I was excited about having a house on a safe, quiet cul-de-sac, a place with a big back yard and a basketball hoop for what we hoped would be a growing family. I was also certain that working together on a home that we could call our own would make our marriage stronger. It would be ours together. It would surely bring us closer.

Once in our new home, we had weekend barbecues with good friends that we met in our church and we planted one of those beautiful umbrella trees in the front yard. I brought rocks down from my family's cherry orchard to landscape our gardens. We put in a nice lawn and a sprinkler system. With all of our hard work, it was a beautiful place to live. I was proud of what we had created together. Our house was a home. Everyone in the neighborhood had young children, it seemed, and Scott made good friends just as we did. It was all so much fun, and I envisioned our happily-ever-after right there in that house.

It wasn't to be, though. Dave hurt his back, so he could no longer work as a welder. As he was forced to look for other types of employment, our income dropped. I hung onto my job at the dentist's office and continued scrambling to earn extra money doing odd jobs.

It wasn't enough. Unfortunately, we had spent money foolishly. We got so caught up in making everything perfect, that we bought without thinking about the consequences. For instance, we wanted the yard in right away, so we did the landscaping and installed a sprinkler system and paid for it with a credit card. We bought a big screen TV and stereo on credit, too. In short, we wanted all of the things that go with owning a house—without having to wait and save for them. We lived on credit when we should have been pinching pennies to make things work.

We hadn't prepared for a situation like this. We began falling behind on our house payments. Finally, we went to several different credit consolidation companies to see if they could help us manage our bills so that we could stay in our house. They couldn't help us. We had dug ourselves too deeply into debt. There was nothing else to do. It was time to see a lawyer and declare bankruptcy. We lost our house and my car, a bright red Pontiac Grand Prix with tinted windows — that I probably never should have bought in the first place.

We were bankrupt and didn't have anything to show for how hard we had worked all of our lives. Besides being a huge financial blow to our credit, this was humiliating and emotionally devastating for both of us.

What was worse, our beloved, former home sat empty for a good long while after we moved out of it. I would drive by it sometimes and cry when I saw our poor house vacant and abandoned-looking, the yard rapidly becoming overgrown with weeds.

"Oh my gosh," I'd think as I drove by, tears streaming down my face. "Nobody is taking care of my yard, and I worked so hard on that." All of that hard work, and it was all gone.

I had thought life was difficult before, with our marital and financial struggles. Now it felt like things were over and we might never be happy again. I was completely overwhelmed and terrified.

*

The only way you can survive when something catastrophic

happens in your life is to keep putting one foot in front of the other, especially if you have a child to raise. My parents were about to serve a mission for our church and offered their home for us to live in while they were away, so we moved into their house with Scott. We were so grateful.

It was hard for Dave to move into my parents' house and I appreciated that; however, we were both relieved as well as thankful to have a roof over our heads. At least we weren't on the street. We took Scott out of his school in Clinton and put him in preschool in Pleasant View.

The transition back to my hometown was comforting for me, because I was back in my childhood sanctuary. I knew all of the neighbors and even some of the teachers who were still at the school. Our ward was great, too, about welcoming us back, and I was happy to begin serving there.

Dave, on the other hand, appeared to experience a sense of failure because he felt like he hadn't provided sufficiently for our family. He attempted to go back to Weber State to earn his degree—his workman's compensation package paid the tuition—however, he didn't finish. It wasn't until many years later that he confessed he quit going to classes at night because he was afraid that I wouldn't be able to handle Scott on my own at night. Although that didn't make sense to me it still made me feel inadequate as a mother at the time.

By the time my parents came back from serving their mission for our church, I was finally pregnant for the second time—after nine years of trying! Scott was as excited about the baby as I was; he had been praying for a brother or sister for years. He even asked me to come to show-and-tell at school, where he proudly showed his classmates an ultrasound picture of "his" new baby in my belly!

I weighed close to 200 pounds when I got pregnant that second time, which meant that I was heavy; however, people weren't rolling their eyes at me just yet. I gained 50 pounds during the pregnancy, though, and that weight pretty much stayed on after I had our second child, a beautiful girl that we named Annie.

Being heavy again didn't mean that I stopped being social. I was the fun-loving, reliable friend everyone could count on. My patients in the dental office loved my calming manner and gentle hands, so much so that many of them would schedule appointments specifically with me or stop by to visit even if they were just passing by. I was the person in the neighborhood who other people knew they could count on if they needed a ride or any other favor.

I was active in our ward, too. The main organizations (called auxiliaries) of an LDS ward, overseen directly by the bishop, are the Relief Society (the LDS Women's organization), the Young Men and Young Women organizations, the Primary (the children's organization), and the Sunday School. Members like me serve in different areas of our wards; in my case, I was asked to help in Primary as a teacher. Scott and I had a lot of fun baking cookies or brownies for the neighbors in our ward on Sundays as another form of service as well.

I volunteered at Scott's school, too, helping with class parties and bake sales. I was always smiling and making friends everywhere I went. I even became a room mother for Scott's class. My role in the class was to help out by arranging parties and helping the teacher in any way she needed me.

I smiled on the outside. But on the inside, I was growing ever more miserable. I always felt insecure going to Scott's elementary school because I wasn't one of those skinny, cute moms. I would weep at home before I went out, because I had nothing to wear. I would get so frustrated shopping for clothes since nothing fit. I had just three or four outfits that I would rotate through over and over again.

Meanwhile, I put on my happy face as an accessory to go with everything. The last thing I wanted was for other people to know the depth of the desperation I was experiencing behind my smiling, friendly facade.

*

Just before Annie was born, we moved out of my parents' house and into a little, red-brick, rented house across from the elementary school.

Dave can be very helpful. For instance, he is the first person to help out if someone's car breaks down by the side of the road, and we were lucky because our landlord loved the fact that Dave was always willing to help him out fixing machines or doing other odd jobs. That really helped whenever we fell behind on the rent.

We were both relieved to be in our own place again. Also, it was so much fun to finally have another baby, and a girl at that! I loved dressing my baby girl and fell completely in love with her. That was easy to do, since Annie had such an infectious, friendly personality—even as a baby.

That was a good thing, too, because things didn't get any easier after Annie was born. My health suffered dramatically during those postpartum months. I tried again to breastfeed and failed even more miserably than before. I even had one of our neighbors, a lactation specialist at the hospital, come to help me multiple times, yet I failed over and over again to breastfeed. This time my nipples became separated and had to be reattached. I developed a breast infection that turned into a severe staph infection, leaving me reeling with fever and so weak that I could barely pick up the baby to change her diaper.

I was fortunate that my mother and sister, Lesa, lived so close by. They did all they could to help me out, and I was finally able to get through those first difficult months and be well again.

Meanwhile, our financial situation was not improving. Dave and I were the poorest we had ever been, always struggling to pay our bills. I still, to this day, have a little anxiety attack when the phone rings, because bill collectors were always calling our house and threatening us whenever we owed money. There were often notices coming in the mail or taped to the front door saying that our electricity or telephone service was about to be shut off. I felt as though I were living on the edge of a cliff with a sheer drop to ragged rocks below.

From the little rental house, we then moved into another house that we could call our own—sort of. My brother's wife called one day to say that they wanted to buy a farmhouse on four acres as an investment property, and she wondered if we might consider renting it. This was a small, pale yellow brick farmhouse located about a mile straight up our hill on the mountain in a nice neighborhood.

This seemed like the break we needed, both financially and

emotionally. Dave was keen on the idea of living on a farm. He grew up in Salt Lake City, so he's a city boy; however, since he went to Montana on his mission, Dave discovered that he had a real love for farming.

For my part, I was excited to be living near my brother, whose own house was just around the corner from our modest farm. There was a beautiful, gated community nearby and we'd have children around the neighborhood to play with our kids. We were excited about getting the kids involved in 4H and being part of a new ward. We moved just before Thanksgiving, and Dave and I felt the tension ease between us, despite having to rely on the generosity of our ward for help with groceries and on my sister-in-law for a Christmas tree.

We began to acquire animals when we moved to the farm. Scott, and later Annie, raised pigs for 4H; we also added another dog to the pair of dogs we already had, plus a flock of chickens, which lived in a coop that Dave and the kids built. Our yard and driveway were a maze of bikes and scooters, and neighborhood kids flocked to our house because it was so much fun there. Living there felt like a fresh start for all of us, especially because I could see that Dave was finally beginning to spend more time with the children. We seemed happier as a family.

You would think that with less stress, I would lose weight, right? Wrong! I continued to pile on the weight. Although I still hadn't realized this about myself at the time, I am an emotional eater who eats whether I'm happy, sad, frustrated—you name it. And when I ate, I always overate; it didn't matter whether I was comforting myself or celebrating.

Our finances weren't much better, either. The blows to my self-esteem kept coming. Fortunately, people in our faith are amazing about offering a helping hand. The bishop helped us with bills, as did my parents; I would mow the lawn or do other odd jobs around my parents' house in payment.

The dentist I worked for was kind, too. When we moved out of my parents' house, for instance, he knew that we wouldn't have a washer and dryer, so he bought them for me. He was generous with bonuses at Christmas, and one year, when my boss knew how much

Scott wanted a bike, he polished up his son's year-old bike and gave it to Scott.

Even with so much help, Dave and I had to continue relying on the bishop's storehouse, which is a market where you can go and pick up groceries that the church has paid for. It was humiliating to have other people know that we were living in a borrowed house and still didn't make enough money to feed our family.

I continued to feel angry that Dave didn't work as many hours as he could or find another job, even one flipping burgers, while I was still working and trying to do things like sell candles on the side. Dave's response to this was that he had watched his father work so many jobs to support their family that he was never home. "I want to be around for our children," he maintained. "I don't want to be an absentee father."

Ironically, of course, this put me in a position where I had to work more hours and spend more time outside of the house away from my children. I didn't feel like I had a choice. I couldn't see any end to our financial troubles and my self-esteem continued to plummet. I wondered if I would ever be happy again.

*

Like most lifelong dieters, I never stopped trying to lose weight, no matter what was happening in my life. Whether I was on the grapefruit diet or the Atkins diet, the cabbage soup diet or Weight Watchers, it seemed like I was doing math calculations on my food all day long. Around 1998, though, I discovered a program that not only made weight loss possible by cutting calories, it could help change your lifestyle completely—mentally as well as physically.

This program, documented in the book *Body for Life* by Bill Phillips, left me feeling optimistic and inspired about weight loss and the possibility of actually transforming my body. I loved the book and everything he had to say. I was so taken by his wisdom about weight loss—and by the before-and-after pictures in that book—that I even drove three hours to hear him speak and asked him to sign a copy of his book for me.

Bill, a former competitive body builder, created *Body for Life* as a 12-week nutrition and exercise program. In 1996, he held the first *Body for Life* Competition, which required competitors to write about their experiences with the program and send in "before" and "after" photos to win prizes.

I was so impressed that I requested a video of the *Body for Life* contest from the previous year. Watching it amazed me. Yes, I admit that winning money by entering that contest appealed to me. Even more appealing was the way the contestants were helping other people change their habits, live healthier lives, and feel better about themselves.

"I'm going to be just like that someday," I told my friends. "Those people who win the *Body for Life* contests are so inspiring. I want to be just like them."

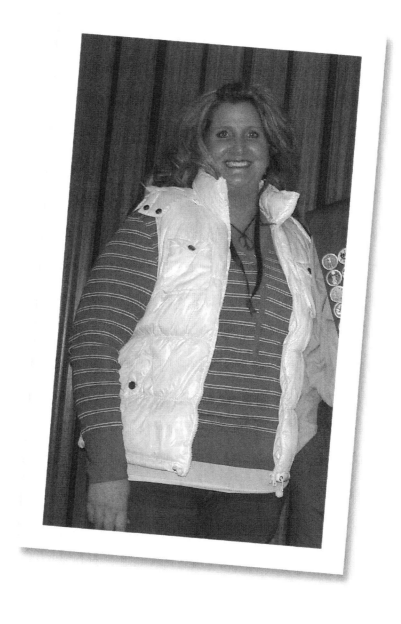

4

YOU HAVE A FAT MOM!

"The human body is nothing short of a miracle—
definitely something to be appreciated and thankful
for every day. Just think of the things your body
allows you to do, to experience, and to create."

— Jill Birth

B eing overweight and constantly trying—and failing—to lose
the extra pounds I'd managed to accumulate through the
years didn't just affect *me*. My yo-yo dieting and emotional eating
impacted my entire family.

While other mothers were running around the block or biking
with their kids, it was all I could do to huff and puff as I climbed stairs
or made it out to the car because I now weighed 263 pounds. It also
meant that my children and I suffered a lot of humiliation.

Once, at a family pool party, I promised my kids that I'd go down the water slide and swim with them—just like all of the other moms and dads. That promise ended in disaster. I got no more than a few feet down that water slide when I realized I was stuck. My hips were literally wedged in the slide because I was so big! The only way I got down was because my nephew climbed up the ladder and slid down, pushing on my shoulders hard with his feet to dislodge my hips enough that I could squeeze down that narrow space. I landed with a whale-sized splash in the water. Everyone laughed, even me, though I was dying inside. I wished at that moment that I could just run and hide.

That was about the same time that my son Scott started feeling embarrassed about my appearance after one of his friends observed—truthfully—that "you have a fat mom!" My poor son loved me—I knew that—although I'm sure he must have felt ashamed that I was so obese that strangers rolled their eyes when I walked—or waddled!—down the street. He couldn't understand why I wasn't thin like his friends' moms. I couldn't understand it, either. What was wrong with me?

I was at the end of my frayed, emotional rope. I was well aware that my eating habits were out of control. First thing in the morning, all I could think about was food and whether I was going to be "good" or "bad" today—even as I searched the cupboards for something that I was convinced would make me feel better. It didn't stop there. My whole day, I focused on when and what to eat.

My food fixation had become a problem in every area of my life, from my marriage to motherhood, from my job to how I served others. I would go to the grocery store, for example, and if there was someone I'd gone to high school or college with who I was embarrassed to see, I would sit in my car in the parking lot, waiting for them to leave rather than risk letting them see what I looked like now.

Around that time, I was on my lunch break from work when another humiliating incident caused me to take stock of my weight and my life. I was running errands, and, of course, I was starving—or felt like I was, because I was stressed—so I went through the drive-thru of a fast-food, Mexican restaurant and ordered tacos to eat while driving back to work. At a stoplight, I was shoving one of the tacos into my mouth when I noticed that the man in the car next to me was shaking his head at me making a face. I rolled down the passenger side window. "Why are you giving me that look?" I called.

"Because I just think it's so disgusting when fat people are driving and eating," he yelled back, then sped away as the light turned green.

Stunned, I finished my drive to work and told my friends what had happened. "Gosh, I'm so sorry," they said. "That was really rude. And mean, too!"

They were right. Yet, in a way, that man's reaction to me was a wake-up call. I finally had to get serious about looking at what I was eating, trying to get the weight off, and getting control of my health.

*

One of the biggest stumbling blocks I faced in losing weight was that I had so many pounds to shed. I'm a planner, always trying to perceive what the future might bring. Whenever I started a diet I would sit down and map out how much weight I would plan to lose in one month, three months, six months, a year. The problem was that if I didn't reach my goals on whatever schedule I had set for myself—say I hadn't lost 30 pounds in the first three months the way I'd planned—I would just lose heart and give up. *What's the point of trying?* I'd ask myself. *You know you're just going to fail.*

How do you go from being an overweight woman who feels unworthy of love to being someone who loves herself? It isn't easy, especially if you're in a relationship with someone who thinks he's motivating you, yet unknowingly criticizes you in ways that pierce your heart just the same.

Nonetheless, with a lot of time spent on my knees praying to the Lord, I decided to try to lose weight again anyway. And, you know what? Sometimes all of the signs are there and point you in the right direction. That's what happened to me.

Around this same time, a patient in my office talked to me about trying a nutritional program that involved both cleansing your body of impurities and substituting some of your ordinary food with extremely nutrient-dense shakes and snacks. This patient had rapidly lost an incredible amount of weight on this program. The quick weight loss while maintaining and building lean muscle mass was what was most attractive to me in the beginning. The results were dramatic. I was interested and excited!

Almost that same week, my friend RaQuett, a nutrition specialist who worked in an Ob/Gyn office and often counseled women about weight loss, openly admitted that she had a food addiction.

"Jill, I think you're addicted to food, too," she said.

I looked at her in disbelief. "There's no way," I said. "Don't be telling me something I don't think I am!"

I didn't think of myself as "being like that," and I was too upset and taken aback emotionally by her stinging observation to own up to being an addict—not yet.

However, I was definitely intrigued by the idea of cleansing my body—something I'd never tried before—combined with supplementing my meals with nutritious shakes. One of the toughest things for me, as I've said, is that I'm an "all or nothing" kind of person. Once I started eating back then, it was always tough for me to maintain any kind of vigilant portion control. Another obstacle that kept me from committing wholeheartedly to any weight loss program was the slow pace. My patient assured me that this new program was fast and simple. I wondered if it could be my ticket to transforming my body—and my life.

At that time, this program required you to do two full cleanse days. Then, for the next five days, you would continue to drink their nutrient-dense shakes, followed by two more full cleanse days. The program was meant to rid your body of impurities; weight loss was only considered a side benefit.

What a benefit! Following this new program, I lost 40 pounds in record time and felt so much better than I ever had before. Besides being thinner, the program was helping me build lean muscle mass, not to mention the fact that I felt amazing and had boundless energy— something I had definitely been missing before.

People started noticing how good I looked and asking me what I was doing to lose the weight. I was happy to share my experiences. It wasn't long before I was sharing information about the program with friends and family.

At the same time, Dave and I seemed to be doing a bit better. It was during this time that I earned a free cruise through the company I had been working for. It was a three-day cruise to Catalina Island and down to Mexico. It was the first time Dave had ever seen the ocean. He and I had never taken any kind of trip like this before—we just never had the money to travel—so it was a lot of fun.

It brought out Dave's romantic side as well. It was during that cruise that my husband did the nicest thing for me that he'd ever done. Long ago, I had lost my engagement ring while I was getting my grandparents' yard ready for our wedding reception. I just looked down and the ring was gone! We tried to find it, but we never did.

On that cruise, Dave presented me with another engagement ring, a beautiful diamond. That was a big moment for us, when he walked me down to the edge of the boat and gave me the ring and kissed me.

I actually got seasick on that cruise—too sick to enjoy the midnight buffets, for sure! However, what I didn't know was that I was sick for a very good reason: I was pregnant with our third child, Zackery. My pregnancy meant no more cleansing. I kept drinking the nutritious protein shakes; however, because I stopped monitoring everything else that I was eating, by the time I gave birth to Zack, my weight had skyrocketed to 265 pounds. Here I was again.

After Zack was born, I knew that it was time for me to take more drastic action. What could I possibly try next?

ILL BIRTH

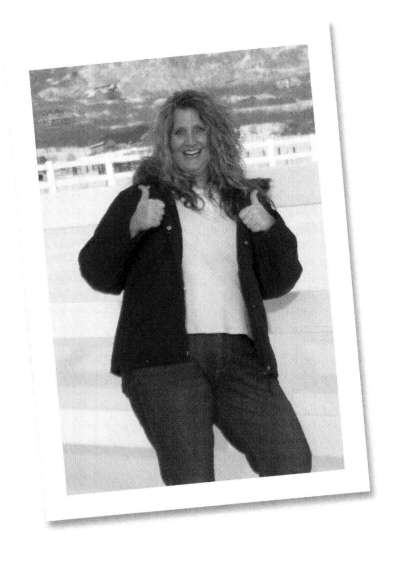

5

THE TURNING POINT

If you are going to fail, fail in motion!
Fail as you stumble on your climb up the mountain.
Fail . . . forward!

— Jill Birth

My sister Laurel had a handle on her recovery from anorexia by college. However, she has always been an exercise fanatic and a careful eater, so she remained thin. My sister Lesa, on the other hand, is wired more like I am and has constantly struggled with being overweight. Any time I went on a diet, I would talk it over with Lesa and ask if she wanted to try it with me. She almost always did, yet her weight issues were so severe that she became depressed and went through times when she hardly left the house and slept all day. Finally, Lesa made a firm decision to get healthy and lose weight. She decided that the only way to suppress her appetite was surgical and had a gastric bypass when she was 36 years old.

Gastric bypass surgery involves dividing the stomach into large and small portions. The small portion of the stomach is sewn or stapled to make a pouch that can only hold about a cup of food. Then the surgeon disconnects this stomach pouch from the first part of the small intestine and reconnects it to the intestine farther down. This reduces the calories and nutrients your body can absorb.

About 10 percent of the people who have this type of surgery suffer complications. Unfortunately, my sister was one of them. She became so sick that she had to have yet another surgery to stretch out her esophagus. Like me, Lesa hadn't yet fully accepted the idea that she was an emotional eater, a food addict who needed to kick that habit before she could become healthy. After the surgery, she continued trying to eat the same way she used to—binging on unhealthy, rich foods—however, that would make her really sick.

I remember one time in particular, Lesa called to talk to me about it. "I feel like my best friend just died, because I can't eat the things I love," she cried. Over the next few years, unfortunately, Lesa gained her weight back. I knew I didn't want to suffer what my sister had. I also knew I had to do something.

At that point the tension in my marriage had finally reached a place where Dave and I had no choice. We had to enter marriage counseling once again. I say once again because Dave and I had been in and out of marriage counseling for years. This time it was a final attempt to save our marriage. When the subject of my weight struggles came up during these sessions, I told the counselor that I wanted very much to start losing weight again; however, I was afraid to reach my target goal.

"Why is that?" the counselor asked.

I swallowed hard, looking at him instead of Dave as my eyes teared up. It was tough, yet I knew that the time had come to tell the absolute truth. I didn't want to ever hide my feelings from Dave again. I admitted that I had reached the point where my marriage was so troubled that I was desperate for the feeling of self-worth that I didn't feel like I was getting from my husband. This didn't make me proud of myself, yet I knew I had to be as honest as possible if I was ever going to recover from what I now understand to be my food addiction and find that confidence and self-esteem I so desperately needed to embrace love, live my dream, and serve others.

I had been unhappy for so long all the while thinking, "Who would want me this way?" In the back of my mind I wondered if I finally lost the weight, could I develop the confidence to finally move away from my marriage? Was it a lack of confidence that kept me with him? "I'm afraid my marriage might end if I ever get thin," I said.

The counselor shook his head. "That's no reason to hang onto your weight, Jill," he said gently. "You don't know that you'd leave your marriage if you were thin. Nobody can predict the future. You need to lose the weight for yourself, and we'll cross that bridge when it comes."

I took a deep breath and felt surprisingly liberated. It felt good to be totally honest. The counselor had given me permission to think ahead to a future where I wasn't so grossly overweight—or so incredibly miserable. How could I go about losing weight this time when nothing I'd tried so far had stuck? I knew that I didn't want to suffer through what Lesa had with her gastric bypass surgery.

Not long after that counseling session, I learned of another woman in town who'd had a successful lap band surgery. A lap band surgery is a simpler and less risky procedure than a gastric bypass, although still pretty invasive surgery. During this surgery, surgeons place a silicone ring around the top portion of the stomach. Depending on how much weight you want to lose, the band is tightened with saline shots delivered through a special port from within the ring. People don't lose weight as quickly with lap band surgery as opposed to gastric bypass surgery; however, patients generally suffer fewer medical complications.

The reason I considered it was because the woman in town who'd had the surgery looked so terrific that I didn't even recognize her afterward, she was so thin. The problem was that our insurance wouldn't cover that surgery, which even at the time could cost upwards of $12,000. How was I going to justify spending money we didn't have for something that I should be able to control? How selfish was I?

I was so desperate to rein in my insatiable appetite that I was willing to go into debt to have an artificial device installed to do it. I started researching medical loans to pay for lap band surgery. Dave, however, was adamantly opposed to the whole idea. "You know you can lose weight on your own," he said. "You've done it before. You don't need some foreign object in your body."

Even our marriage counselor suggested to Dave that he think about it. "Jill really wants to lose this weight," he told Dave. "You might want to consider agreeing to the surgery for her happiness." However, Dave dug his heels in even more at that, showing a stubborn side, which I am so grateful for today. I probably would have tried harder to convince him that lap band surgery was worthwhile if it hadn't meant both of us incurring so much debt. We were barely making ends meet as it was, though.

I would have to do something else. But what now?

*

Once I accepted the idea that I couldn't financially take on the debt incurred to have lap band surgery, I searched for something else that might motivate me. That's when I made up my mind to try out for *The Biggest Loser*.

If you've never watched this television show before, you've really missed out on one of the greatest reality TV shows of all time. This show, which features obese people competing to win a cash prize by losing the highest percentage of weight, first aired in 2004. I had been watching it from that first season and never missed it. I was inspired by the contestants, whose bravery and determination were so honest and awesome.

Each season, *The Biggest Loser* starts with a weigh-in to determine the contestants' starting weights, which serve as the baseline for determining the overall winner. People on the show are then grouped into teams and work out with trainers to exercise and start eating differently. Various challenges and temptations are featured on each show; the people who overcome those challenges and temptations are given special rewards, like full immunity from being voted off the show.

Each week, there is a weigh-in to determine which team has lost the highest percentage of weight for that week. The person who is voted off is the person who has lost the lowest percentage of weight. The team that has lost the lowest percentage of weight during that week gets one member voted off, usually by the other teams. Then, when the number of contestants has shrunk to a smaller number, the contestants start competing one-on-one against each other.

Contestants on the show often lose as much as 10 pounds in a week. I found this both alarming and inspiring. Was that kind of weight loss even possible? Was it healthy? I was determined to find out.

More importantly, I was once again inspired to help people. Just think. If I could figure out how to do this successfully, I could help so many people live longer, healthier, happier lives. I was in!

Part of trying out for *The Biggest Loser* involved making a video, which I then put on YouTube. In the video, I was brutally honest. I outlined my weight struggles and lamented the fact that I had lots of "before" pictures, yet never an "after" picture. I wanted to be as honest as the people I so admired on *The Biggest Loser*. I sincerely put myself out there for the world to see, knowing that I had to be completely sincere and open to be successful. At 263 pounds, I even appeared in a red jogging bra and matching shorts working in the dentist's office and surrounded by cheering coworkers!

The video worked. I think the show's producers could definitely see that I was serious about going public with my struggles. They did the initial interviews with potential contestants in Utah and I made the cut. I couldn't believe it!

Throughout this process, one of the toughest and most surprising challenges was overcoming the doubt and lack of support expressed by my family. Dave flat out refused to say anything on my video. I put in a picture of us anyway, looking almost happy together. My son Scott, who was 16 years old by then, was completely mortified.

"You mean you're going on TV as a fat person?" he asked, rolling his eyes.

I laughed. "How else would I go on TV?" I asked. "I am a fat person. Besides, wouldn't it be great if I finally got skinny and could inspire so many other people? Think of the people I could help."

I drove to Salt Lake City alone for the final interviews. I was so excited, thinking, "Oh my gosh, I'm going to be on *The Biggest Loser*!" I was finally making my dream come true: this show would help me reach my target weight and be more fit, and it would serve as a vehicle for me to inspire others to do the same. I would show them how. I would let them know that they weren't alone.

When I didn't make it onto the show, I was disappointed. I have to admit that it was tempting for me to fall into a pit of despair. Then I decided that God had a bigger plan for me. Rather than let myself be disappointed, I felt that something else was meant to happen. Along the way, I still found it fantastic to meet the judges and other people struggling with their weight. I returned home feeling more determined than ever to continue on this path toward a better, healthier life. Maybe God knew that I had to do this on my own.

*

My friend RaQuett saw this new resolve in my eyes when I came home and said, "Okay, are you ready to try that full body nutritional cleansing program again? Let's do it together."

I agreed, yet this time we decided to do things differently: we would start our own "Biggest Loser" group right in our neighborhood. I had reached a turning point in my life, and I had never been readier to embrace the new challenges ahead.

I decided that I would try the same nutritional cleansing program that I had been successful with before having Zack. I had first started the nutritional program back in 2002, releasing the 40 pounds quickly during that initial attempt to control my weight. When I got pregnant with Zack and gained that weight back, plus more, I became depressed again. I would watch people qualify for the program's 100-Pound Club and become emotional seeing them, because they inspired me so much. I wanted to be up there with them! I knew that the Lord really wanted me up there, too, because I was too self-conscious and uncomfortable with my body the way it was now to be of much service to other people.

One reason the program didn't completely match my needs before was that it had required you to do full-day cleansing, which just didn't fit my mental state at the time. Instead of using the products the way they were meant to be used, I would manipulate the program. I'd binge on my favorite foods, then cleanse, binge some more, and then cleanse again. It was so crazy; some people would look at me and say, "That program must not work. Look at Jill Birth." The program worked all right. I just abused it.

By now, however, the program offered another way to cleanse that I knew I could successfully follow because it allowed you to incorporate small, sensible amounts of healthy food into the program each day. I was also more mentally ready to commit to not just losing weight; I was ready to release the weight forever. I learned from a friend that if I kept trying to "lose" the weight, somewhere in my mind I knew I would "find" it again someday. If I "release" the weight I am committing to letting go of the weight forever. I liked looking at it this way and that is what I did. From that moment on I looked at it as "releasing" weight that I would never "find" again.

I had learned from my previous mistakes. I couldn't let my past failures continue to haunt me. I was determined to succeed this time. I really was ready to transform myself—and my life. I had accepted the fact that I was addicted to food. RaQuett and I started attending 12-step addiction meetings almost immediately. In my heart I knew this would be the key not only to my own success, I would soon be able to help many others achieve theirs as well.

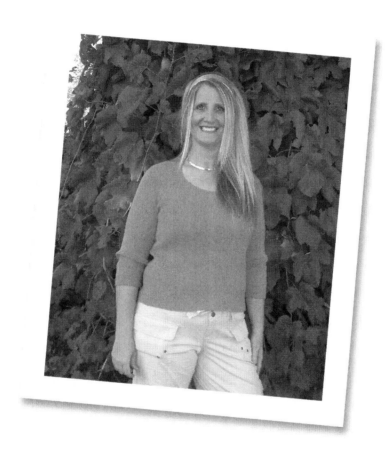

6

STEPS IN THE RIGHT DIRECTION

Faith is taking the *first step*
even when you can't see the whole staircase.

– Martin Luther King, Jr.

There are many kinds of addictions, and every single one of them is tough to beat. However, food is one of the trickiest addictions because it's easier to hide and the toughest to avoid. Everyone needs food to survive, so a food addict is not like an alcoholic who makes a decision to stop drinking alcohol, right? Plus, eating is acceptable and expected—nobody would stop you on the street for eating a cupcake in public the way they might try to stop a drug addict from injecting heroin into his arm.

One of the reasons I was able to stick with this particular program was because I geared myself up mentally for it beforehand. Lucky for me, RaQuett finally convinced me to try a 12-step addiction program. "I think you're addicted to food, and I know I am, too," she kept telling me.

I still got mad at her when she said this, yet I wasn't sure why. I now know I was really feeling defensive at the time. However, the more RaQuett said it, the more I began to realize that there might be something to this. She was right. I still thought about food every minute of every day, whether I was eating or not. So, one day, she and I just looked at each other and said, "Let's go to one of those meetings."

One of those 12-step classes were run by my church and attracted everyone from alcoholics to people addicted to prescription drugs and pornography. Every meeting started out with us sitting in a circle with whomever else turned up, saying our names, and announcing our addictions.

The first time I said, "Hi, I'm Jill, and I'm addicted to food," I felt like people looked at me like I was crazy.

The guy next to me, who had confessed that he was addicted to prescription drugs, shook his head and said, "Food is not an addiction." The thing is, this guy must have weighed about 400 pounds! I just looked at him and felt such compassion toward him, knowing that he didn't realize he was a food addict, too.

The 12-step meetings really helped me start acknowledging how, when, and why I was driven to eat the foods I did. I realized that I wasn't eating to sustain my life or even for the pleasure of good food. I ate when I felt emotional. If I was happy, I would eat. If I was sad, mad, or bored, I would eat some more! It didn't matter if my emotions were bad or good. I needed food to be my best friend. Food was *my* drug of choice.

The first step in recovery from any addiction is admitting that you have one and recognizing what it's doing to your life. For me, one of the most important steps I took toward getting a handle on my food addiction was to tell God that I was powerless and that I couldn't manage this food addiction without Him. "I can't do it on my own, Lord, not even with willpower," I said in my prayers, as I asked Him to put my addiction in His hands every day.

As you work through the 12-step program, you also do an inventory of your life. Just as a business that never takes a regular inventory is bound to go broke, we must do exactly the same thing and take stock of our lives honestly. This is a sort of ruthless fact-finding mission. First, we search for the flaws in ourselves that might have caused our failures, so that we can face the truth of our situations as we prepare to turn ourselves over to the Lord for help. Where have you been? Where did your addictive behavior start, and how far did you go with it? Where has that behavior led you?

As we search through our past behaviors and take a moral inventory of ourselves, we can sort through the chaos of our lives to discover who we really are. This is an important step in ridding ourselves of the burdens that have weighed us down in the past.

After doing that inventory, you admit these flaws to God as well as reading it to someone else. I read mine to RaQuett and she read hers to me. Then we decided to burn our inventories as a way of saying that we weren't going to let whatever happened in our past lives hold us back from achieving our goals any more. (This step is what I now call a "Burn Letter," and I'll go over that later in the chapter called "Clean Your Slate.")

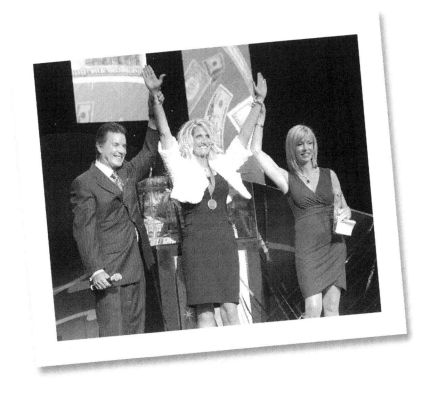

7

THE BIGGEST WIN OF MY LIFE

If you want to fix what is broken,
if you want to fix YOU, start by loving yourself—
every single piece of you!

— Jill Birth

With the help of the Lord and the 12-step program, I signed up for the Transformation Challenge that the nutritional company I still worked for was offering—a contest offered in which the winner achieves a total body transformation. I liked the idea of working toward something as well as the accountability. It suddenly got exciting to think that I could not only release my weight and get fit, but I could win a contest at the same time!

Whenever I wanted to cheat or manipulate the program, I would rely on my 12-step program as well as remember the fact that I was meant to do something greater. I was going to figure this out and, someday soon, I was determined to inspire others to do the same. I watched *The Biggest Loser* faithfully and played right along with the show at home, in my *own* way: I released weight not by working out six to twelve hours a day like they did, but by working out maybe four hours a week and following the new, modified version of the same nutritional program I had used before Zack was born. I had to do this in a way that would allow me to be successful.

I did not cheat. For the first time, I used the products exactly the way they were meant to be used. I followed the program to the letter. This time there was no manipulation whatsoever. I did exactly that, and only that, for seven months—the length of *The Biggest Loser* season—and the weight was really coming off. It's amazing what happens when you follow a program designed to give you better health!

What kept me going? Why didn't I cheat this time, the way that I had every other time? One key difference was that I now had lots of support. The 12-step program was there for me any time I needed it. The women in the dentist's office who had helped me make my video for *The Biggest Loser* were still cheering me on, as well as my family and friends. My friends in *the Biggest Loser* group I'd started with RaQuett were right there, too, journeying forward with me towards our common goal of becoming healthier.

RaQuett and I had put together this Biggest Loser group somewhat selfishly, because we knew we needed lots of support if we were going to release weight. We were friends who otherwise were apt to cheat together! Being in this group gave us additional accountability—not because we were afraid that the members in this group might judge us, but because we knew they were counting on us. Another inspiration that motivated me was Kim Olson, one of the first people to release 100 pounds using the very program I was doing. I was so happy for her. Someone else had done it. If she could do it, I could too.

I was determined to be that same inspiration to others that the people on *The Biggest Loser* television show had been for me. During our local Biggest Loser group meetings, we spent one hour at the beginning of every Thursday night's meeting doing a mind-body-spirit class to put everyone in the right frame of mind to release weight. First we began with 20 minutes on the mind focusing on visualizations, including vision boards and affirmations, which I discuss in detail in the second part of this book.

Next, we spent 20 minutes on the body, doing exercises, like lifting weights, and drinking water. Finally, we concluded our meetings by spending 20 minutes on the spirit, talking about the 12-step addiction program because this program taught me how to recognize the real reasons why I ate.

We didn't care if group members were using the nutritional program that we had so much success with or following some other plan. We just wanted to create a safe haven where people could work together and feel accepted.

At our Biggest Loser meetings everyone would weigh in, chart their progress, and put a dollar in the pot for attending the meeting. *The Biggest Loser* for that week went home with the pot of money; some weeks it was a lot, when as many as 80 people might show up! At the end of the evening, we'd crown our own Biggest Loser and take a picture. I loved it that the meetings kept us all accountable and moving forward—including me! We all looked forward to seeing each other get smaller, happier, and more confident! It was wonderful.

*

Just like many of the members of our Biggest Loser support group, I, too, was battling my own food addiction. This was when I decided to write *my* own burn letter. This letter described all of the incidents I could remember that had involved food in some emotional way—many of which I've included here in this book—along with my honest account of why I thought I had become a food addict and attempted to destroy my body, my life, and my dreams by overeating.

After I read the letter aloud to RaQuett, I burned it over her kitchen sink. Putting my past behind me was a crucial step in my recovery. Only by recognizing the path I'd taken to this place, accepting it, and forgiving myself for the past, would I be able to move forward.

I also, with RaQuett's help, created a vision board. I'll talk more about how you can do your own vision boards later in the book. For me, this was a simple poster board where I tacked up inspiring quotes and photographs to keep my motivation up and my resolve strong. For instance, I put up a picture of a really fit woman who was out running, because I had always fantasized about someday completing a marathon—despite the humiliation I'd suffered as a fat little girl who the gym teacher kept yelling at in class.

The vision board didn't just help me imagine the possibility of releasing weight or running a marathon; it even helped with my marriage. Dave and I were struggling again after tragedy struck our family. Right after Zack was born, Dave's mother was killed in a horrific car accident—with his dad driving and my kids in the car. Thankfully, the rest of them were fine; however, Dave was so upset that he completely withdrew from me emotionally. He was inconsolable in his grief and it broke my heart.

At one point, I went to RaQuett, brokenhearted and sobbing because Dave had become a different person. I felt as though I wasn't able to comfort him and was worried. He seemed lost. She said to use my vision board to affirm the changes that need to take place, whether they were about making my marriage stronger or being thin. "Put your dreams out there like a prayer to Heavenly Father," she said. "Tell Him the specific things you want." Hearing her say this made me remember a favorite saying of my friend Lenny Evans: "God adores me and is anxious to give me all that I will receive." I needed to remember that God wanted me to be open to receive His blessings.

I followed her suggestion, and, you know what? I started looking at my vision board as a living, breathing thing I could continue to add to as a way of supporting a positive vision for my future—and for my family's future. For example, when I used my vision board in the way RaQuett suggested, I realized that Dave needed more than me to get him through this dark time and that my place was to be there for him when he needed me.

Besides the burn letter and the vision board, another thing that kept me moving toward my weight goal this time was a really good bathroom scale. I bought one of those scales that calculate your weight in pounds and ounces as well. Now I could look at my success every day, see that I was another two or three ounces down, and know that I was headed in the right direction. I charted every ounce lost by writing down what I weighed each day on a paper I kept by my scale. I celebrated every ounce lost!

By the season's finale on *The Biggest Loser* in December 2010, an amazing thing had happened: I had released 100 pounds! Not only that, I had lost a higher percentage of weight than any other female contestant on the TV show. And don't forget—they were exercising many hours a day, while I was working out only three or four times a week.

I felt a huge sense of accomplishment. For once, I was proud of myself. I had reached deep within my own soul to find the courage and confidence I needed to pursue a goal and reach it. I had learned how to ask for the right kind of support and I had received it. I had finally done the work and had been completely honest with myself. I was at peace knowing that I now understood what it took to get here. The honesty, the soul searching, and the support—it had all come together. I was excited to realize that I had finally figured it out and couldn't wait to share it with anyone in the world who had been where I had been. I knew I could not keep this to myself.

*

Because RaQuett and I had lost weight so successfully and felt great, we were happy, healthy products of the products! People I went to school with, family members, even complete strangers were coming to us now to regain their health. These weren't just overweight or obese people, either. Some just wanted to cleanse impurities out of their bodies. Some were athletes looking for ways to build lean muscle and improve their performances on the track, field, or court. We began sharing what we had learned and these wonderful products with others. It was so exciting to help so many people that my heart was full of gratitude. We were giving them hope and they were realizing their dreams. It was fantastic.

My transformation still was not complete. I started my second body transformation challenge right after Thanksgiving. In January,

I went with RaQuett to a 2011 kickoff event for the nutrition company we'd been representing. While we were there, we saw last year's winner of the Transformation Challenge. She looked amazing. I was so happy for her.

This contest, we found, isn't just about weight loss—it's about a total body transformation. For instance, one of the contestants lost 28 pounds *and* completely transformed her body so that her muscles were completely ripped and defined. What I learned later made it even more exciting. A person representing the company announced that there was going to be a big change in the 2011 Transformation Challenge: instead of taking home $10,000 for the grand prize, the winner would take home $120,000!

RaQuett and I grabbed onto each other. "You're going to win that stinkin' challenge, Jill!" she said.

And, you know what? Right then, the Holy Spirit spoke to me and said, "You can do this. You have it in you." My resolve was solid—grounded in His belief in me, my belief in myself, and what I wanted for my future.

I was ready to compete. I was going to win that title and make my lifelong dream of inspiring other people to become fit and healthy come true at last. I knew winning the Challenge was going to require dedication and commitment. I was excited. I now had the clarity and certainty to do it. I was confident that I would be successful.

*

I went right home and got to work. Now that I had this huge goal, I mapped out my strategy. I knew how much weight I wanted to release—my goal was to release half of my original body weight of 263 pounds, which was where I had started with the first challenge 24 weeks before. That meant releasing another 31 pounds. Not only that, it meant that I needed to get fit. Really fit. I needed to plan out my exercise strategy as well as my food intake. I could do this. I *would* do this.

I decided that one of the first things I'd do would be to put my dream out there on my vision board. I tacked up all kinds of inspirational sayings and pictures. And then, looking at that picture of the lean girl running, I decided to sign up for a half-marathon. I printed off a program called "Couch Potato to 5K" that I found on the Internet and began following it. This seemed like the easiest and most affordable way to release body fat and build up the lean muscle I needed to truly transform my body.

Gradually, I started running instead of walking, pushing myself at first to go from one mailbox to the next, then picking out more distant landmarks as I started running a little more every day.

At the same time, I stuck faithfully to my nutritional cleansing program. The program had become easy by now because it was so familiar *and* I felt great doing it. I had a shake for breakfast, a healthy meal, a shake for dinner, and then drank the cleanse juice. Eventually I worked up to full cleanse days and continued to follow the program exactly.

I mapped out this plan day-by-day and submitted it—and myself—to the Lord, saying every morning, "Heavenly Father, I'm asking you to allow me to put my eating and food addiction in your hands today."

I knew that meeting this challenge successfully would mean progressing one day at a time. If you do things one day at a time, you can conquer almost anything! I'm living proof of that. Plus, I had already discovered that the only things I could control were how much I exercised, what I put into my mouth, how good a mom I could be, and my relationship with the Lord. With that knowledge and confidence, I knew that I could accomplish anything.

Instead of eating a special treat as a reward for releasing weight, I also came up with a list of rewards that were designed to make me feel good without allowing me to weaken my resolve. For instance, I had my first pedicure when I got down another 10 pounds. I posted my progress on Facebook, too. I got support from all over the world telling me how good I looked and encouraging me to keep going. I was not alone.

In addition, I decided to keep a journal. Doing that was, without a doubt, one of the single most important steps I took toward becoming more aware of my eating habits and how those habits were linked to my emotions. I literally wrote down what I did to exercise, every bite of food I ate every day, and how I was feeling at the time in my food journal. Putting these things together helped me understand what triggered my eating.

Because I wrote down not just what I ate, *as well* as the feelings I was having as I ate that particular snack or meal, there was no longer any way for me to disguise the fact that my emotions were deeply tied to when and what I ate.

I readily admit that this was a tough exercise for me. I found it difficult to be completely honest—even with myself! Sometimes I'd cheat and just "forget" to write down something like a handful of cookies grabbed before dinner or that second helping of pasta. Again, I was manipulating the program, and as a result, I was sabotaging my own success.

Gradually, though, I got a grip and forced myself to make a serious, detailed account of my eating habits and exercise. I had to be completely honest—with myself. It was the only path to success. Keeping this journal forced me to think about what I was doing moment-by-moment. It was a tool to help me become more aware and mindful of what I was feeling as well as how I was living. In the process, I was learning a great deal about myself.

What I discovered by doing this really and truly shocked me. For instance, I was eating practically a whole second dinner while I cooked dinner for my family, just by sampling the foods as I made them! Eventually, the journal helped me rein in my appetite; often, I would choose not to eat something because doing so would mean having to write it down! Accountability is powerful.

By May 15, I'd done it. I had cut my body weight in half—from 263 pounds to 132 pounds. I had decreased my clothing size from a size 22 to a size 4! I was fit and ready for that half-marathon. I was never prouder of myself than I was on the day I crossed that finish line. I had achieved so many things that I never could have imagined accomplishing when I was a child. I had learned to manage my demons and get truly healthy. Shoot, I had even become a half-marathoner!

A mere five days later, I had my "after" pictures taken, or what I like to call my "photo shoot." This was fun and exciting—a far cry from the days when I used to hide if anyone took out a camera because I was so embarrassed by my size.

Then I put everything together—a 500-word essay, my photos, and a video—in a package to send in for the Transformation Challenge competition and waited with fingers crossed and many, many moments on my knees. I knew in my heart that, even if I didn't win the contest, I had won in a much more important way, by gaining my health and learning a way to help others achieve what I had achieved for myself.

*

Right before the end of my challenge I went to the company's spring event. Everyone was amazed by my transformation. People were so happy for me. At the beginning of the event, the person on stage addressing the crowd suddenly said, "I just want to recognize someone here today, because I haven't seen her in a long time and she has totally transformed herself."

When he announced my name, I was shocked! I was sitting right in the front row. What could I do, but go ahead up there on stage? Me! The person who was once too afraid in high school to deliver an oral report, and the same girl who quit her public speaking class in college because she was so self-conscious about her weight! It was exciting and surreal at the same time. This moment made me face the fact that, win or not, I had done it. No more hiding or trying to escape who I was. I was there, transformed into my new self and living my new life. I now knew what it took and I was ready to share it with the world.

The Challenge finalists were announced in July. They called me at work; I couldn't answer the phone because I was with patients. "We have some good news for you!" they told me when I finally had a chance to return the call. "You're in first place in your category!"

I told all of my patients and the girls in the office the news. Boy, that was a happy moment! We were all yelling and screaming. I broke down in tears, it was all so surreal. "Oh my gosh, I really won first place!" I'm so happy!" I said over and over again. My heart was pounding with excitement. Winning first place in my category meant that I would now be among the finalists eligible for the grand prize of $120,000 and the title of "Grand Prize Champion!" If I could win, this could be my way to inspire others on a grander scale!

Once my mom found out that I was one of the first-place contestants for the Transformation Challenge and that I would have a big gala dinner to attend, she took me shopping for what I call my first "prom dress." This was such a special moment for me. I had been so overweight throughout high school that I'd never been asked out by a boy to a prom or any other fancy occasion, so we decided to make the most of the moment. She and I shopped until we found the perfect dress: a fitted, floor length, deep pink gown. It was so beautiful! I couldn't believe that was me in that gorgeous gown. With my new body and my new dress, I really did feel ready for the prom at last.

*

The Grand Prize celebration was held in San Diego in August. During this event, every finalist had to appear before a panel of judges; that panel would ultimately vote on the winner. Even though I knew I was first in my category, I also understood there was no guarantee that I'd win the Transformation Challenge. I'd heard so many other stories of amazing contestants that I knew any of the finalists were worthy of that prize. Deep down, I knew that we were all winners.

When I arrived in San Diego for the celebration, I was excited. My anticipation had built to a nearly unbearable degree, yet it was heightened even more by multiple photo shoots, one right after the other. Everything felt surreal as people attending the event kept approaching me, excited to meet me and shake my hand or hug me. I loved every minute of it. I had no idea that so many people had been following my progress on Facebook or had watched my YouTube video—the one I'd made for my Challenge portfolio and decided to post myself, which apparently had gone viral.

I was excited by the attention. It was so heartwarming to hear people say, "You've inspired me so much, Jill. I love you," "You lifted me up," or, "You made me feel like I can do this, too!" One woman even showed me a picture of her baby daughter that she'd named after me! It was all amazing and so much fun!

As these words of affirmation continued to flow in my direction, I was held aloft by the support of many well-wishers in a way that made me realize the magnitude of what I had accomplished. I really was the kind of inspiration to other people that I had always hoped to be. My true success was assured. Win or not, I was determined to keep inspiring and helping others.

Dave flew down on Sunday with the kids to help support me—something I really appreciated, since we had been going through so much hurt and pain together for so long. I wanted my kids to see their mom up on stage and hopefully be proud and grateful that I had accomplished my goal. That meant the world to me! My parents, sister, and nieces drove from Utah to California to cheer me on as well.

At last, the moment arrived for my interview with the judges; however, nothing went quite as I'd imagined it would go. I had planned my interview with the same careful attention to detail that I had used in planning my weight loss and exercise, writing everything out beforehand so that I would be fully prepared. However, when I arrived early for my interview, I discovered that the finalist who had been scheduled to be interviewed first by the judges still wasn't there.

"Jill, you can be the first one," they said. "You can go ahead in and talk to the judges now."

At that exact moment, I had just put one of the program's yummy chocolates infused with green tea extract in my mouth! These always make me feel good, although now I had chocolate all over my teeth as I was smiling at the judges! Can you believe that?

In a way, that was probably the best thing that could have happened, because it definitely broke the ice. When I started laughing, the judges did, too—especially because I had brought my size 22 pants with me, and I was able to show them how I could now fit my hips and both of my legs into one leg of those pants!

From there, it was easy to talk to the judges about my journey to transform my body—and myself. I knew that this was the start of my happily-ever-after and I was excited to begin the next chapter of my life. I did not even try to hide my enthusiasm!

"Whether I win the grand prize or not," I said, "I know that I've won either way. I feel amazing. I have my health and confidence back."

The interview felt very organic, like a comfortable conversation. My excitement came from a special, genuine place. Although I felt that it went well, I still wasn't convinced that I would be chosen as the grand prize winner.

Finally, though, the big moment arrived. When my name was announced as the winner of the Transformation Challenge, I felt like I'd won the Miss America Pageant. When I told the story about climbing the mountain with Scott, the audience became just as emotional as I was in telling the story. I was so excited and happy that I didn't even notice the streamers being shot up into the air as part of the celebration until after I saw film footage of the event.

It was the biggest win of my life—so far. Reaching my personal goal wasn't about winning money or releasing weight in the end. It was about knowing that I had worked hard to accomplish a goal I had been dreaming about for so long. No more humiliation, no more shame. I had addressed my food addiction. I could hold my head high, and my kids saw it all.

I had finally crossed the finish line. By releasing half of my body, I had won my life back at last. Now I could begin to live my dream of helping others. I could not wait!

PART 2: YOUR STORY

The only person you are destined to become is the person you decide to be.

— Ralph Waldo Emerson

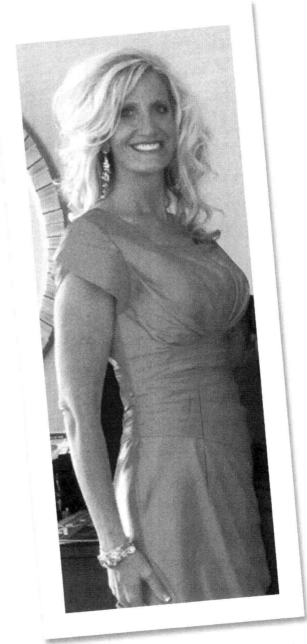

My first "prom" dress.

INTRODUCTION

Now that you've read my story, it's time to tell your own—a story where you're in charge of your own happily-ever-after ending!

It might seem to you that I have ended my journey with a complete transformation of my body and my life. Yet, in fact, this is a journey without end. Getting into recovery for my food addiction and, in doing so, living my dream is something I take one step at a time every single day. I couldn't have done it without the help of my friends, my family, and the Lord, who supported me every step of the way and took over when I was too weak to make it on my own. There were days I literally made it through my own transformation on my knees, in prayer. And day-by-day, it became easier. I felt myself changing inside and out.

I promised the Lord that this was His victory and I would absolutely remember that every single day. In keeping with that promise, I want to pay forward my own good fortune by helping you with your own intimate battle. However you wish to transform your body and your life, I am here to help guide and support you. May God bless you in your journey to find the courage to be the person He has always intended for you to be, the person I *know* He can absolutely help you become!

Together we can do this, using the simple, step-by-step strategies I have outlined for you in the second part of this book. Believe in yourself, even if only a little in the beginning. Watch that belief grow into determination, and blossom from determination into passion. There will be no stopping you!

Happiness is not something
you postpone for the future;
it is something you design
for the present.

— Jim Rohn

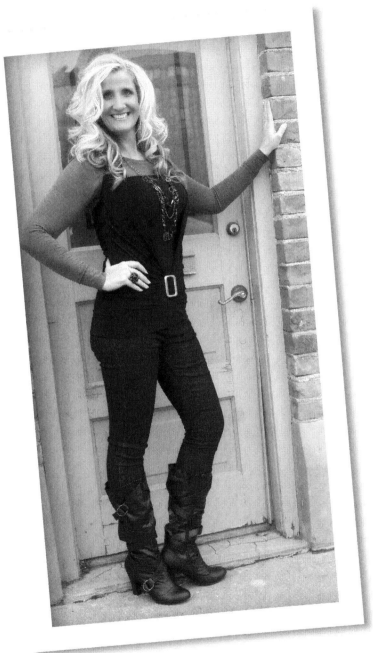

100 pounds released!

8

NO MORE EXCUSES!

The thing you want to do least is probably the thing you need to do most.

— Jill Birth

Throughout most of my life, I tried everything to "lose" weight, taking "before" pictures 24 different times, each time saying to myself, "This time I'll do it." I failed every other time, continuing my weight battle and not addressing my food addictions, continuing to be ashamed and watching my confidence and self-esteem plummet.

If there is an excuse out there for not being able to release weight, believe me, I've heard it. In fact, I have probably even used it myself! Before you start on your own body transformation so that you can live your dreams, let's just get those excuses out of the way, okay?

Here are some of my favorites—and what you can tell

yourself if you try making this excuse instead of cleaning your slate, starting your life over, and living your dream the way you were meant to.

"I Don't Have Time to Plan Healthy Meals"

We're all busy. Most of us have to balance work, family, and home responsibilities in ways that we never imagined, working 12-hour nursing shifts or stopping off every day to check on an elderly parent, working two jobs to put ourselves through school, taking care of young children, or doing farm chores. I told myself that I was too busy to plan meals, too, especially after having children and trying to balance work and home chores. How many times did I zip through a fast food restaurant at my lunch hour because I didn't take the time to pack a nutritious lunch? I shudder to think!

The truth is that it's easy to eat healthy foods—it just takes a little advanced planning. Here are a few tips: Go to the grocery store and get pre-cut veggies if you don't have time to dice and slice your own. Cook the week's meals ahead of time on the weekends and freeze them. Stock your pantry with healthy nuts and other high protein snacks instead of cookies and chips. Keep fresh fruit and veggies in the fridge at work as well as visibly at the front of the fridge at home so that when you open that door, you see those options first.

All of these tips can help you make healthy food choices to maintain your appropriate blood sugar level. After a while, buying and eating healthy foods will become a habit and your go-to snacks, I promise!

"Good Food is Too Expensive"

I definitely had this mentality for a while. Healthy food doesn't really cost more than food that's poor in nutrients. Think about how much you spend on a bag of chips, then look at how many apples you can buy for the same price! Also, if you're addicted to soda pop and telling yourself "it's only diet soda," think about the chemicals in those drinks and add up the cost of a case of soda a week. That money can buy a lot of vegetables! In general, you want to stay away from the prepackaged foods in the center of your grocery store and shop the outer aisles (dairy, meat, fruit, and vegetables) to eat healthier foods and save money.

One last thought: healthy food is a long-term investment in your health, so it's worth a little extra money to eat a nourishing diet. It will be cheaper over a lifetime to eat healthy foods than it would be to battle health problems associated with obesity, like heart disease and diabetes, later on.

"I'm Too Old to Release Weight"

People in our society think it's normal that, as we age, we're just going to weigh more and suffer from chronic illnesses like arthritis. We're supposed to just accept it.

The truth is that you don't have to suffer aches and pains or other degenerative diseases simply because you're older. You live longer if you weigh less, according to most related research studies, and releasing even a few pounds can make a huge difference in how you look and—more importantly—in how your body feels. You're never too old to release weight and feel better! I am living proof that, once you cleanse your body of impurities and flood it with nutrient-dense foods, your body has the ability to go from acidic to alkaline, from inflamed to calm, from aching and holding onto excess weight to working well and releasing that excess weight, allowing the body to heal itself the way God intended.

"I'm Too Tired" or "I Don't Have Time to Exercise"

This is one of the most common excuses I hear. It's also one that I have often used myself. There was a time when I would sleep late every weekend morning because I couldn't bear the idea of getting up. I was so depressed about my weight that I would even take naps during the day! It's true that if you've been eating poorly and you're overweight, you're going to feel too tired to even walk around the block. That certainly happened to me!

As you eat healthier foods and cleanse impurities from your body, you'll feel invigorated. And, even if you start very gentle exercises, like push-ups against your kitchen counter or leg lifts in front of the TV in the privacy of your bedroom, you'll start to feel like doing a bit more each day. The more exercise you do, the more you'll notice that your endorphins kick into gear—those are the natural chemicals in your body that give you that feel-good bump in energy. This is especially true if you exercise outside. A body in motion stays in motion!

In regard to finding the time to exercise, fit it in during your day. Park far away from the mall entrance. Take the stairs instead of the escalator or elevator. Sit on an exercise ball at work instead of a desk chair. The point is that you can fit it in if you choose to. You don't have to start with an hour each day, just start. Develop the mindset that you will do some sort of exercise every day. Then as you start to add to it and do more, schedule that time for yourself like an appointment. Care enough about your health to make it a priority.

"I Have Too Much Weight to Release"

Uh huh. That's a good one. I've used this excuse myself many times—remember: I had over 100 pounds to release when I first seriously started my own life transformation! I would get prepared to start a new diet and feel so excited thinking about the "new me." Then, a week into it, I'd be starving and miserable, and it would all seem too overwhelming for me to keep going, because I thought it would take me 5 years to release the weight at the rate I was going.

"I might as well just quit," I'd tell myself, as I reached for whatever package of cookies was handy in my cupboard.

The thing is, sometimes weight really does come off an ounce at a time, and that's fine. Get one of those scales that measure in ounces as well as in pounds, and celebrate every ounce lost. I'm not kidding! Make small goals—visualize releasing 5 pounds, then 10, etc. Your brain is a powerful tool when it comes to visualizing what it will look and feel like when you reach your goal! Please, take me seriously. It really does make a difference.

"It's Not 'Magical Monday' Yet"

Ah, "Magical Monday." You know what I'm talking about! How many times have you waited for a certain Magical Monday after a big weekend to declare the start of a new diet? Because I worked with a lot of other women in a busy dental practice, we were always coming in on Monday and deciding to try a new diet because we felt so guilty about how much we'd been eating over the weekend. Or I'd talk with my sister or my friend Shelly, and we'd set a goal of "the day after New Year's" or "the day after my birthday" to try some new way of "losing" weight. And, you know what happened? We'd binge big time before that magical day, therefore starting five pounds over where we were when we declared the diet! There is nothing magical about any particular day. Just start right away!

"I Don't Want to Give Up My Favorite Foods"

We all have our "go to" comfort foods. For some, it's that soda pop mid-morning or the ice cream we eat just before bed. For others, it's that sour cream on the baked potato or butter on our toast in the morning.

There is a "good" way to eat. There is a "better" way to eat. And there is the "best" way to eat for optimal results. You have to start by looking at where you are and what you want. If you can just toss out a couple of things on your usual list of rich foods—maybe salsa on a baked potato instead of butter and sour cream—and make those adjustments a few at a time, you will release weight without feeling deprived.

Just keep asking yourself, "What is my goal weight really worth to me? Is it worth sacrificing that goal to eat these potato chips for a snack?" You'll be surprised by how strong you can be when you keep your goals uppermost in your mind! Remember, it's all about progress, not perfection, when you're transforming your body and your life. Do what you can to remind yourself why you started your weight loss journey in the first place.

"I Can't Do This Forever"

In fact, you can eat healthy foods for a lifetime. Many people do. Once you make that mental switch from accepting that you're a food addict to getting a handle on why you eat and become a healthy eater, you'll be amazed at how little those low-nutrient foods you once craved tempt you at all. As you cleanse impurities out of your system, it will get easier and easier to reach for an apple instead of the bag of chips or the cookie jar on the counter, because your mind will be in the habit of craving different things. You'll become mindful of what your body is *needing* instead of what your emotions used to crave.

Eating healthier foods isn't a temporary fix. It's a lifestyle—one that you will love once you embrace it, because of how much better you'll look and feel. You will want it for yourself. Trust me when I tell you that you have no idea how poorly you were really feeling until you fill your body with the good nutrients it has been craving. It's amazing

"So What's Your Excuse?"

Okay, you've heard some of my favorite excuses. Now, what's yours? Write down every excuse you've ever made for why you haven't released weight. Then write down the reasons why this excuse doesn't make sense—even if you have to ask friends and trusted family members to help you determine the flaws in your own reasons for hanging onto those extra pounds that aren't just weighing you down physically, they are weighing you down emotionally, too!

Be honest. You're worth it.

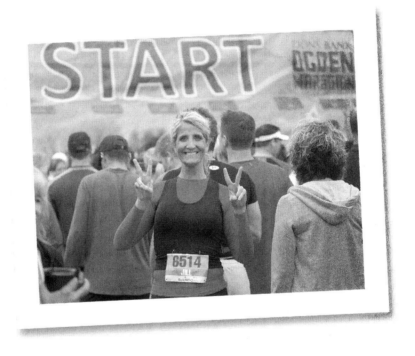

9

CLEAN YOUR SLATE

You are on the path of rising every time you fail
and refuse to be stuck in the failure.

— Jill Birth

During the first part of this book, I told you my story as honestly as I knew how. The thing you need to remember most about my story is that I had 24 starts, 23 fails, and 23 decisions to try again. I know that I'm not alone, and you aren't, either. I'm here for you, just as other people were there to support me when I was where you are now.

It took me a long time to honestly see the patterns I had developed and to understand why I became so addicted to food that my addiction began to control my life. I shared my story with you because I was able to let go of the past and live my dream. I hope to inspire and help you to do the same, so that you can start living your own happily-ever-after as a thinner, fitter, healthier, and happier person.

Taking the steps you need to clean your slate and succeed in transforming your body and your life will require courage, determination, and lots of support from people you trust. As you've seen from my own story, it will mean looking at all of the different pieces of your life from childhood on, so that you can see when and why you began turning to food for comfort. Go back as far as you can remember and try to catalog your childhood and friendships, your intimate relationships and your marriage, your career and your fears, and, yes, your hopes, too. It will be an emotional and eye-opening process, yet it's a necessary step in understanding yourself.

The thing is, right now you probably only see yourself as a failure because you haven't succeeded yet at your goal of being fit and releasing weight. What if your goal is to never lose the desire to win? If you continue nourishing that desire along the way to moving closer to your goal, then you have succeeded!

Even my weight loss attempts that *didn't* result in me weighing even a pound less than when I started were valuable, because these attempts built my character and kept me learning and growing. Each diet really did teach me some golden nugget of information that I needed to add to my treasure chest of knowledge that would ultimately lead to my success.

The desire to win at all costs—to win in the face of all setbacks, to win when winning was laughing at me to my face, to win when I finally caved and bought a few clothes in the next size up, to win when I found myself right back where I started with my last attempt—through all of that, I hung onto my desire to win my battle with food and transform my life. I still had my dream and never gave it up.

That desire to win carried me through failures, defeats, setbacks, personal struggles and losses, lack of support from those around me, and even the voices in my head that reminded me that I had not yet won the battle. And, because I never lost my desire to win, my entire journey was a success! It was worth all of the trials I had endured. I now know that I had to go through this growth process in order to learn how to succeed myself and, hopefully, to inspire others.

For you, it's important to understand how you got to this point in your life, because then—and only then—will you have the self-knowledge about your own journey, so that you can see yourself as a winner and use even your past failures to become a stronger person and get closer to your goal of living a healthier, happier life.

Write Your Own Burn Letter

This is the time to tell your own story. The best way to do this is to write a burn letter—a story you'll write and read to someone you trust, the Lord, and yourself. It can be a letter, a list, or a journal chronicling your thoughts. Write it in a way that's comfortable for you. I'm going to ask you to think back to your parents and siblings, to your greatest accomplishments and humiliations, and to all of the relationships that have worked or failed. Think about how your weight has affected your life—all of it: friends, family, confidence, choices, personality, events, consequences. Everything you can remember!

To get yourself started on this very important burn letter, find a quiet place and time to answer the questions below. Then add whatever you like as you write the letter. I want you to prayerfully consider what events, words, opinions, etc. have filled your life's backpack with stones that you have continued to carry, refused to let go of, and ultimately have weighed you down for years. Write them all down. This is a valuable inventory of your life up until this point.

Don't worry about grammar or chronology. Just use the questions to prompt your memories. Go at your own pace. Answer a few of them a day, if you like, until you feel like you've told your story and put it all out there in black and white. Prayerfully address each question. Leave no stone unturned. The point is to write down your thoughts as you ponder your life and recognize the voices inside that have been holding you back from reaching your goals in any area of your life, whether that area is your weight, career, relationships, or whatever.

What are your earliest memories of childhood?

Would you describe your childhood as happy? Why or why not?

Did you suffer any abuse—physical, sexual, verbal, emotional, or otherwise?

Who were you closest to as a child?

What kind of house did you live in?

Did you have a bedroom to yourself?

Do you have memories of comforting yourself with food? If so, how?

Do you have memories of comforting yourself in other ways? How?

Did you ever eat more than your share of cafeteria lunches? If so, why?

Did you hoard food in your bedroom or any other secret hiding place?

Were other people in your family overweight?

What was the attitude of other people in your family towards heavy or obese people?

When did you first consider yourself overweight?

Did you like elementary school? Why or why not?

Who was your favorite teacher, and why?

Who was your least favorite teacher, and why?

Did you like middle school and high school? Why or why not?

Who was your favorite teacher in middle school or high school, and why?

Who was your least favorite teacher in middle or high school, and why?

Were you ever on a sports team? Did you like it?

What's your favorite memory of high school?

What's your most embarrassing memory of high school?

What was your greatest joy as a young adult?

Did you like having your photograph taken?

Did you ever diet in high school or as an adult? List your diets here, and think about why they worked—or didn't work.

What kind of dating life did you have after high school?

If you didn't gain weight until adulthood, write down when that was and why you think it happened.

What are your best personality traits?

What are your worst personality traits?

Who has betrayed you in life?

Who have you always been able to trust?

If you're married or living with a significant other, describe that relationship. Is it a positive force in your life?

If you're in a relationship that makes you unhappy, list the things you want to change.

If you don't think the relationship you're in now could ever make you happy, why do you stay?

Do you suffer from joint pain, arthritis, backaches, wheezing, or any other health issues associated with being overweight?

Do you have a job you enjoy?

Do you have friends at work?

Do you socialize outside of work?

What would you like to change about your career?

What would you most like to change about your personal and professional relationships?

How would your life change if you lost weight, ate healthier foods, or exercised?

Is there anything you avoid doing because of your weight or body image?

Once you've written out the answers to these questions as well as any other thoughts that may come up as a result of reflecting on your past, hand write your letter in whatever format you choose. Don't type it. There is something very therapeutic about the writing process—trust me. (See "Write Your Burn Letter in Five Easy Steps.")

When you have completed it, I want you to read the letter aloud to yourself first. This is an important step, because it means that you're owning your past and are ready to let go and move on. You are telling the truth here, and only the barest, most uncomfortable truth at that.

Next, read the letter to someone who won't judge you—someone who accepts you for who you are right now, even if it is solely to God. This exercise of sharing your letter verbally helps you put these life events behind you.

Then, once you've acknowledged these things in your life that are both positive and negative, I want you to burn the letter. That's right. Stand over a fire pit in your back yard, the fireplace in your living room, or even the kitchen sink, with a lit match, and set that letter on fire. You are burning the past and all of the negative associations that come with it. (Please do this safely!) The act of burning the letter is so powerful. It is the physical act of letting go of your past. It's like telling Heavenly Father that you are done with your past and you are ready and choosing to move on to greater things!

As you watch your words of the past burn, let them go! Forgive and forget! *That includes forgiving yourself.* Start with a clean slate and begin redefining who you are based on what you deserve!

This is the beginning of your transformation. You are not the person who wrote that letter any more! You are transforming yourself so that you can live your dreams, and letting go of the past is an important first step. You are on your way.

Write Your Burn Letter in Five Easy Steps

1. Think about how your weight has affected your life. All of it: friends, family, confidence, choices, personality, events, consequences.

2. Write these things down. Start with your childhood if you can go that far back. You don't have to write in chronological order.

3. Read your letter to yourself.

4. Read your letter to someone you love and trust.

5. Burn it!

Face Up to Your Food Addiction

I was lucky. I had my friend RaQuett working hard to help me realize my food addiction. I finally faced up to it. Every day she told me that I was addicted to food. Every day I denied it. How could I be addicted to food? It wasn't like food was a drug! Right?

Wrong. The truth is that food can act very much like a drug, altering your body chemically and making your mind crave more of that same salty or sugary taste that makes you think you feel better. In some cases, food addicts trying to break the habit claim to experience both physical and emotional withdrawal symptoms such as headaches, insomnia, mood changes, tremors, cramps, and depression. It's not the food. It's all about how and why you go to it.

Food addiction is real. And, like any other addiction, a food addiction is all about seeking control in situations that feel out of control. Food addicts rely on this comfort to feel less anxious in social situations, to console themselves during anxious or stressful situations, or even to "celebrate" when they're happy.

Food addicts like me worry all of the time about food, weight, and body image. We can compulsively eat abnormally large amounts of food even when we understand that this behavior isn't good for us. We especially tend to crave and eat foods that are harmful, like fatty, sugary, or salty foods. There's a rush involved as you put this kind of food in your body. You know it's terrible for you to be eating the way you are, but you think you "need" it to make you feel better. Yet you never do. Never!

I do understand this cycle from personal experience. We're not alone, either—there are over 18 million food addicts in this country alone! It's a tough addiction, as I've said before, because food is everywhere. Everyone accepts the fact that you're going to eat, and even overeat, in a way that people would never accept you doing heroin, say, or drinking a bottle of whiskey every night. Food is a sly addiction, because we need food to survive and it is around us pretty much every hour of every day. So instead of learning to live without it, you actually have to learn to live *with* it!

The first step to recovery with food addiction is admitting to having the problem. How do you know for sure that you're addicted to food? Here are some common signs. See if any resonate with you:

You think about food constantly during the day.

You feel like you "need" it during certain situations.

You compulsively crave certain types of foods.

You waste more than half of your daily calories binging on unhealthy foods.

You worry about your weight and body image.

After comforting yourself with food, you feel sick, guilty, or depressed.

You repeat the eating patterns that make you feel bad about yourself.

You want to stop eating, yet can't.

You find yourself trying one diet after another and always fail.

You binge and then vomit or take laxatives to purge what you've eaten.

You eat differently in private than in front of others.

You eat to escape your feelings.

You eat when you're not hungry.

You go through periods of fasting, then binge.

You hide food to make sure you have "enough."

You're driven to exercise excessively to control your weight.

You obsessively calculate the calories you've burned against the calories you've eaten.

You often feel guilty or ashamed about what you've eaten.

You're waiting for your life to begin "once you lose the weight."

Do You Need a 12-Step Program for Your Food Addiction?

Food addiction is absolutely one of my greatest challenges in my lifelong pursuit of weight loss and balance because I'm an emotional eater. And when I fall, I fall big! I used food as a drug.

During my own transformation period, I was able to manage this food addiction only with the help of a 12-step program in addition to the support of my friends and my own personal communication with the Lord, who supported me and took over whenever I was too weak to make it on my own. There were days that I literally made it through on my knees in prayer until, day-by-day, it became easier as I felt myself changing inside and out. Know that, even now, it is something I am mindful of each and every day.

So what is a 12-step addiction program, and could it help you? There are many 12-step groups that deal specifically with food issues, such as Food Addicts Anonymous or Overeaters Anonymous. There are others that you may find through your church or another community center that are like the one I went to, which was a 12-step program for people with all different kinds of addictions. Trust me, there's a common bond. On some level, addiction is addiction. Regardless of your vice, you think you are using it to manage your life, when in fact your life has become unmanageable because of your addiction.

Whatever group you choose, it will follow the same principles as Alcoholics Anonymous. The 12 steps are a set of emotional and psychological steps you need to take to help you recover from your addiction. The first step is to admit you have a problem, and the second step is to believe (no matter what your religious affiliation) that a power greater than you can help you with that problem. You don't have to call it "God." You can call it "a higher power," the "universe," or whatever. The important thing is to believe that there is a power greater than your own out there. Personally, I call this power "God."

Most of these groups do not have a professional therapist heading them up; instead, there will be people in different stages of recovery attending the meetings and helping others who are just starting on their personal journeys, because doing so helps them stay focused and strengthens their own sobriety. Hearing others speak with great honesty will help support your own recovery journey.

One benefit of these 12-step programs is that they are free. There are also a lot of them. For instance, about 6,500 Overeaters Anonymous groups meet each week in over 75 countries and have approximately 54,000 members worldwide. There are also hundreds of Food Addicts Anonymous meetings in the United States. Also, both groups have many telephone and Internet meetings per week.

Other advantages abound. Twelve-step groups seem to have the best track record for long-term weight loss and recovery. You are also in charge of your recovery in the sense that you decide what you need to work on. You deal with your addiction at your own pace and have support while you're doing it so that you don't feel so alone, and your shame and past humiliations begin to heal. And, if you need help along the way, you simply ask for it.

There are also excellent group guidelines that will make you feel safe, like "no cross talk," which means people do not interrupt, comment upon, or refer to someone else's sharing. You are not required to share. I will tell you that when you are ready, sharing without interruption, in a safe place, helps you find your voice. Finally, many sponsors (experienced members) are available for phone calls, sometimes every day—no waiting around for an appointment with a therapist when you're feeling low! They can support you and talk you through some tough times.

Best of all, 12-step programs help you deal with the emotions and behaviors that have been fueling your addiction while giving you the tools you need to deal with the problems in your life that have led you to this place and may be keeping you there. It's not about the food. It's about how you use the food to manage your life.

What are the 12 Steps?

These 12 steps are from Food Addicts Anonymous and the LDS 12-step program I personally followed. Note that while these programs use the word "God," these groups are typically inclusive of any faith and of people who are agnostic or nonbelievers as well. The steps are similar to the 12 steps you'll find in any 12-step recovery program from any addiction.

Personally, I wondered why the steps are written in the past tense if it was something I was beginning, knowing it was a process I would need work through. I also wondered why it was written as "we" as opposed to "I." At the time, even though I was doing it with a friend, I knew the journey was mine alone. When Alcoholics Anonymous, the organization responsible for creating the 12 steps, decided to record the steps they took to achieve their sobriety for others to follow, not many understood the concept or believed it possible to achieve such a state of management over their addiction. The steps are written in the past tense to show that each step was followed in order to achieve sobriety. Additionally, the steps are written in plural form to show that it was done together as opposed to doing it alone. This is a very important concept. Isolation can often lead to a relapse for the addict. By agreeing to follow them, we:

1. Admitted we were powerless over our food addiction—that our lives had become unmanageable.

2. Came to believe that a Power greater than ourselves could restore us to sanity.

3. Made a decision to turn our will and our lives over to the care of God as we understood God. (In the LDS version, you decided to turn your will and your life over to the care of God the Eternal Father and His Son.)

4. Made a searching and fearless written moral inventory of ourselves.

5. Admitted to God, to ourselves, and to another human being the exact nature of our wrongs. (In the LDS version, you admitted to yourself, to your Heavenly Father in the name of Jesus Christ, to proper priesthood authority, and to another person the exact nature of your wrongs.)

6. Were entirely ready to have God remove all these defects of character.

7. Humbly asked God to remove our shortcomings.

8. Made a list of all persons we had harmed and became willing to make amends to them all.

9. Made direct amends to such people wherever possible, except when to do so would injure them or others.

10. Continued to take personal inventory, and, when we were wrong, promptly admitted it.

11. Sought through prayer and meditation to improve our conscious contact with God as we understood God, praying only for knowledge of God's will for us and the power to carry that out.

12. Having had a spiritual awakening as the result of these steps, we tried to carry this message to food addicts, and to practice these principles in all our affairs. (In the LDS version, your spiritual awakening is a result of the Atonement of Jesus Christ.)

Don't Forget Your Mind-Body-Spirit Connection

There are profound spiritual concepts embedded in any 12-step addiction program that are meant to help you forge a stronger connection between your mind, your body, and your spirit. For instance, the spiritual principles listed in Step Twelve of *The Twelve Steps and Twelve Traditions* of Overeaters Anonymous are the following (with the LDS version in parenthesis if it's different):

Step One:
Honesty

Step Two:
Hope

Step Three:
Faith (Trust in God)

Step Four:
Courage (Truth)

Step Five:
Integrity (Confession)

Step Six:
Willingness (Change of Heart)

Step Seven:
Humility

Step Eight:
Self-Discipline (Seeking Forgiveness)

Step Nine:
Love for Others (Restitution and Reconciliation)

Step Ten:
Perseverance (Daily Accountability)

Step Eleven:
Spiritual Awareness (Personal Revelation)

Step Twelve:
Service

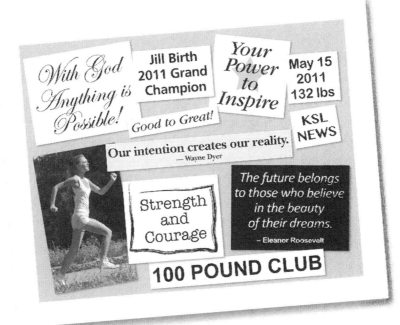

1 0

CAPTURE YOUR VISION

There is a reason for everything you do.
Understand those reasons, and only then
can you change the outcome.

— Jill Birth

As I said earlier in the book, my friend, RaQuett, was the one who first inspired me to make a vision board. She instructed me to go home and put together a poster board with sayings that inspired me, photographs that represented my future goals, and affirmations about who I was—and who I would choose to become. "Just hand your dreams and your visions over to the Lord, and trust in Him," she assured me.

When I put together my first vision board, I weighed 263 pounds and the idea sounded completely nuts to me. You know what?

I did it, and it worked. One by one, my dreams have come true!

Make Your Vision Board

I will be very honest with you, creating my vision board was scary at first. What it meant was for me to envision what I believe I really *deserve*. It meant that I had to step past the fear and realize that I am worthy of what I am asking for. I struggled with that. Who am I to ask for such extraordinary things? Then I read an amazing book by Jack Canfield called *The Aladdin Factor*. It taught me that the act of asking was my first step in taking action. In asking my higher power for what I *deserved,* I was taking a necessary step in reaching my destiny and realizing my vision for my life. If I didn't take this crucial step, I wouldn't command it into my life. Simply put: If you don't ask for it you won't receive it.

If I could wave a magic wand over your head to give you the power to do anything and be anything you wanted to be, what would you wish for? Put the answers on your own vision board. Put on it *all* of the goals you have in mind, not just releasing weight or living a healthier life, include all of those dreams you have. What kind of life would you want to live, if you could do anything at all? It's not up to you to worry about how these dreams will come true. Just put the dreams out there for now and see what happens. Dream big!

Do you want to take your kids to Disney? Take a romantic cruise with your husband? Buy a new car? Do you want to go parasailing or swim with dolphins? Do you have a dream of walking through tulip fields? Put those things on your board, too! Too many people live every day the same way, getting up to go to work (if they're lucky enough to have jobs), then coming home to care for their children, put dinner on the table, and watch a little TV before bed. Is that what you want?

Is that all that you want? Or, if you could have anything at all, would you choose to have bigger, more exciting goals for your life? What words come to mind? Come on, keep going! Write down the trips you want to take, the business experience you've always wanted to have, the relationships you seek with your friends and family, even the kind of place you'd like to live in during your retirement.

What about "freedom" from the trap those extra pounds have created, "confidence" to wear a bathing suit or go to a family event you used to be so self-conscious at that you couldn't enjoy it? What does it look like to feel confident? What does it look like to feel like you have all that you desire? Where are you? Who are you with? Don't limit yourself in any way. Think of a life full of abundance. Come on . . . DREAM!

Vision boards help you identify and voice your dreams and goals. Once you have done that, it will be easy for you to seek and receive help in making your vision a reality! You can create a vision board out of a poster board, a presentation board, a plain old piece of cardboard, etc. After writing down all of your goals and dreams, find images, words, and quotes that represent each item in magazines, newspapers or online. Cut them out and glue them onto your board. Keep in mind that the more specific and detailed you can make your visions, the better the board will work for you!

Hang your vision board where you will see it before you go to bed at night and again when you wake up in the morning. A friend of mine even took a picture of hers and keeps it on her smartphone as well as in her purse so that it's available whenever she needs that reminder of what she is working toward. In fact, my kids and I put little glow-in-the-dark stars around each of our vision boards so that if we get up during the night, we have the opportunity for yet another reminder of what our vision is for our lives.

At the beginning of each day and before you go to sleep, spend five minutes going over the details of the board in your mind, because that's when your subconscious mind is most readily available to visualize your dreams and goals. Use all of your five senses to visualize living the life you have placed on your vision board. Envision specific experiences you want to have. How does it look, feel, smell, sound, and taste to you? If it's a new car, what does it look like? See yourself sitting in the seat with your hands on the steering wheel. What does it feel like? What does it smell like? Feel the leather seats beneath you. The more specific you can be about your dream, the closer to reality it will become.

It's fun to teach your kids how to make their own vision board and you can even make a family vision board. It helps you all dream about what your visions and goals are together. Recently, my kids and I made one. When we were all finished, I asked my kids if they had everything on the vision board. My daughter said "just a sec" and ran off to the computer. After a few minutes she returned with a picture of a girl on her knees scrubbing the floor. I asked her to explain what the point of the picture was and she smiled and said, "I'm choosing to have my own maid!" We all chuckled and glued it on the board.

Do not reason away your vision. The point of making a vision board is to help you start dreaming so that the universe can find a way to open up and help you reach your aspirations. Although your conscious mind will kick ideas out if they seem irrational, your subconscious brain will get excited about the possibilities of living a full, rich life where there are no barriers. You'll be amazed by the visions you can create for a better life—and at how your dreams will start coming true in unexpected ways! Don't forget what I said before. If you don't ask for it you won't receive it. So don't be *afraid* to ask; get excited! You are taking your first steps toward realizing the future of your dreams. Be specific and **dream big!**

Easy Steps for Making a Vision Board

1. Think about it before you begin. Really focus and take some time.

2. Start by writing your visions on paper.

3. Put your specific dreams and goals on it.

4. Don't hold back! Put down all that you want for yourself.

5. Search magazines and the Internet for images, words, and favorite quotes that represent your visions. Draw or write what you're looking for if you can't find it.

6. Pin or glue your visions onto poster board or a bulletin board.

7. Take imperfection action. What does that mean? Don't think it has to be perfect to begin using it. You can always add to or change it at any time.

8. Put the board where you will see it often—in your bedroom is ideal. You might think about putting a picture of it on your smartphone, too! Do whatever you need to do to have it in front of you when you need it.

9. Visualize your dreams and goals for five to ten minutes before you go to sleep and when you wake up each morning.

Affirmations to Live By

In addition to creating a vision board (or many of them, like I have), write out some affirmations that are unique to you and your life. Once you've written them out, post them in various places around your house. Every time you see one of them, stop and read it aloud. Eventually, these affirmations will become part of you, and will give voice to the self-esteem and confidence you need to meet your goals for transforming your body and your life.

Always start each affirmation with positive, active phrases like "I am," I deserve," "I have," or "I choose" rather than "I can" or "I want." I learned from reading *The Success Principles* by Jack Canfield to choose to act "as if." Act "as if" you are already that positive, confident person. If you say something like "I want" or "I need" then you will always want and need because you are talking as if you haven't realized your goal yet. Speak as though you are already successful in that area of your life.

Living "as if" is actually fun as well as very powerful if you take it seriously. When *The Success Principles* came out, I attended a party where we were asked to dress "as if." The party was filled with people dressed in amazing attire that showed who they were going to be. The party was lots of fun, but you know what? I felt empowered. That was when I realized that it really was going to happen. So, please do take living "as if" seriously. You will move closer to what you are creating on your vision board even faster!

I write some of my affirmations on my bathroom mirror with a dry erase marker, so that I can have them in front of me every day. Just to give you some ideas of what these might look like, here are a few of my own affirmations:

With each pound released and reduction in size, I know I am releasing negative connections to my past.

I am in the light and a powerful light. I stand in my truth and I am in love with myself.

I always know when my kids need me, what they need at the time, and that they are loved.

I am spiritual and intuitive.

I have all that I require to live the life of my dreams.

I am creating the body of my dreams.

I am on purpose.

I choose to see the good in others. In doing so, I see the beauty in myself.

I am the author of my own success story.

I take full responsibility for my life and my actions.

I choose to be happy every day.

I love all that I am.

I choose to acknowledge all of my successes.

I choose to create an abundant life.

My life is amazing!!!

I am the person God intended me to be.

Write a Letter to Your Future Self

Here is another important step to help you visualize how you will transform your life. This letter is to the *you* of your future. See this as your vision board in letter format. Start by picturing your life five years from today. What will you want the *you* of the future to look like? Where will you live? Who are you with? What do you do for a living? What are your friends like? What do they say about you?

How will you create this life? If money, logistics, and responsibilities were not an issue, who would you be? Here are some thought-provoking questions and ideas to help you write that letter to your future self:

Do you want to spend time at the park with your grandchildren?

Will you run a marathon with your son?

Will you travel? Where and with whom?

Will you have a large circle of friends or a small circle of very close friends?

Will you pay forward what you learn?

Will you be more involved in your church or some other kind of service?

Will you devote service to underprivileged children?

Will you give a substantial donation to a charity of your choice?

Are you healthy and fit? Describe yourself.

Are you smiling?

Are you closer to God?

Are your relationships improved?

Have you any regret?

Have you crossed things off your bucket list? And if so, what are they?

Have you realized your dreams?

After you've answered those questions, come up with a detailed description of the life you will have five years from today. Write that description in letter format to yourself. Make it special: maybe write it on beautiful stationery and frame it. As with your vision board, keep it in a place where you will remember to read it often.

Life involves passions, faith, doubt, and courage. The most difficult part of any life's journey is deciding on the destination. Wherever you decide to go in the future—with your weight and all that it impacts in your life—go with all your heart. By creating this letter, you can live one day at a time and in the present moment while reminding yourself of the future you are in the process of creating for yourself!

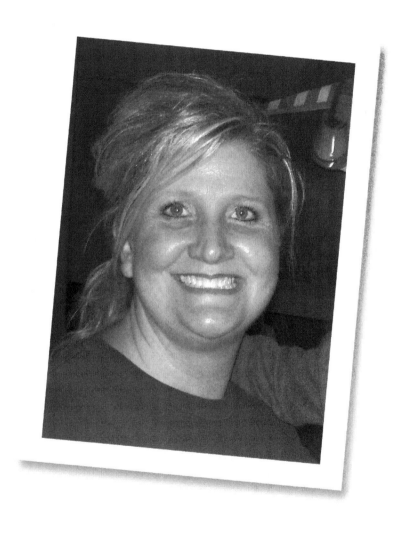

11

LEARN TO LOVE YOURSELF

Love who you are, *right where you are*
on this journey.

— Jill Birth

In the extraordinary movie *Hugo*, the main character is a small boy whose father fixed machines. They were fixing one together when the father died. After this, the little boy said that he would often go to this huge window and look out over the city of Paris. "I'd imagine the whole world was one big machine," the boy said. "Machines never come with any extra parts, you know. They always come with the exact amount they need. So I figured if the entire world was one big machine . . . I couldn't be an extra part. I had to be here for some reason and that means you have to be here for some reason, too." Later in the movie, the boy says, "Maybe that's why a broken machine always makes me a little sad, because it isn't able to do what it was meant to do. Maybe it's the same with people. If you lose your purpose . . . it's like you're broken."

As I watched this movie, I thought about our own human purpose in this big world, and about how, if you don't understand how much there is to love in the world, you lose your purpose. Then you're broken, too.

To fix what is broken inside you means fixing that ability to love. People, like machines, come with exactly what we each need to fulfill our own purpose. If you aren't seeing that in yourself, you are missing something you cannot afford to miss any longer. The first step to learning how to truly love others, appreciate your body, and transform your life is to learn how to love yourself.

I know that's been said a million times, like something we should all know from birth. You know what? I missed that memo. I never realized until going to an intensive therapy workshop in gorgeous Washington state last fall that happiness can only come from within. Nobody else can make you feel happy, or even content. No one. A favorite quote that I recite over and over in my mind is this one: "Happiness is not determined by what's happening around you, but rather what is happening inside you. Most people depend on others to gain happiness, but the truth is, it always comes from within."

All along, I had been certain that it was my marriage making me unhappy and that my extreme sadness over my failing relationship with my husband was causing my food addiction. The truth is that, just like Dorothy in *The Wizard of Oz* had the ability to click her heels and go home any time she wanted, I had the ability to make myself happy all along. In fact, I was the only one who could truly do that, by loving who I was.

I was able to forgive Dave for all of the past hurts once I realized that. Being able to forgive him allowed me to move forward in my life and achieve my goal of releasing weight and fully embracing all of the riches that life has to offer. Forgiving myself gave me permission to truly appreciate all the riches.

Loving yourself isn't always an easy job. If you've been struggling to release weight without managing to achieve that goal, chances are pretty good that you feel like a failure right now. So how do you go from feeling like an unworthy, overweight person to a worthy person who knows that she is winning simply because she is still searching for a way to live her dream?

The answer lies in learning to accept yourself unconditionally, warts and all. You must accept that you are only human. Like everyone else, you have made mistakes. (Guess what? You'll probably make more mistakes in the future, too!) No matter what has happened to you in the past, no matter what mistakes you've made or how many times you've failed in your life, you must forgive yourself and say to yourself that you are worthy of love. Try to think of yourself as the child you once were, and speak to yourself as if you are that child, with love and understanding.

I did that. I remembered how, when I was in third grade, I was the only girl in my class who didn't get invited to a particular girl's birthday party. I was devastated when this classmate said that the reason she didn't invite me was because, "You're too fat and you don't have any friends."

If I could go back in time, I would put my arms around eight-year-old Jill and say, "You know what, Sweetie? You're going to struggle with your weight for many years. Someday you'll release that weight and then you'll inspire millions of other people to find the confidence to live the life of their dreams as well. It will be a full and happy life. You are a child of God. We are all meant for greater things than this."

I can't go back in time physically. However, emotionally I sometimes do, remembering that hurt child inside myself and comforting her with this new knowledge and experience I've gained over the years.

You can do the same thing. You can confront your own past and forgive your own mistakes and the hurts that others have imposed upon you. To do this, you started by writing a burn letter. Now you must write the opposite of what was in your burn letter, replacing that negative view of the events in your life with something positive.

Start with a List: 100 Things I Love About Myself

Once you have successfully written and burned your letter describing all of the things that have held you back, it's time to prepare yourself to move forward and start dreaming again! In this exercise, you're going to write a love letter to yourself. Before you begin the letter, I want you to first write up a list of all of the things you would choose for people to remember about you whenever they think of you.

Next, consider the moments in your life when you have felt the happiest and most fulfilled—the times when you have really used and developed your talents. What were you like during those moments? Were you a leader? The person who cheered on others or made a joke to lift someone's spirits? Did you reach out a helping hand to someone who was struggling?

Write all of those things down, too. I want you to have a clear idea about what you'd choose for other people to see about you, as well as the gifts God sent you here to contribute to the world in the first place. Let yourself freely brainstorm and write down your thoughts as you ponder your life and reflect on the moments when you were at your very best. Take time. Dig deeply!

Got all of that down? Great! Now I want you to keep going! In fact, I want you to list 100 things you love about being you.

Yep, you read that right: 100 things. Not 10. Not 50. Not 99. I want you to write down 100 things you truly like about yourself! These can be major personality traits, like your sense of humor or the fact that you're a movie trivia expert. Or they can be the smallest details that perhaps only you notice about yourself. ("I love my toenails," I wrote at one point, for lack of anything better to say.)

How Do You Write 100 Things You Love About Yourself?

1. Start with things you like about yourself. This can be anything: eyelashes, laugh, personality, etc.

2. Think about what others seem to like about you.

3. Remember compliments others have given you.

4. Ask people you trust this question: "If you had to say five things you like about me, what would they be?"

5. What do you look forward to or feel great doing?

6. Dig deep. Look at *everything*! Include appearance, how you handle yourself at work, integrity, and other personal values. Nothing is off limits!

Write Yourself a Love Letter

Identifying 100 things you love about yourself may seem daunting at first. Put your list someplace where you can see it and add to it often. Keep it with you if you have to. As you continue to seek and develop a loving relationship with yourself, you will find it easier to recognize the infinite number of beautiful gifts that God has given you that make you so unique and loveable.

Once you have your list, I want you to use it to write a love letter to yourself. Think about how you would write a love letter to someone you love. Take the time. Be thoughtful and caring. Write beautifully on special paper if you like. Make it a true love letter that you can cherish.

The purpose of writing a love letter is to help you move past what you are "looking" at in the mirror so that you can start really seeing your own beauty. Doing this will help you remember what makes you such a unique, wonderful, amazing person—no matter what size you are at the moment, you will really learn to love yourself right where you are.

Do a Personal Health Analysis

Are you really such a poor eater? Do you get enough exercise?

While you should have a physical exam by your health practitioner before starting on any serious change in how you eat and exercise, you can do a personal health analysis that will take just a few minutes— and will help you acknowledge the truth about how you look and feel. It's your starting point or, as I like to say, your "current reality" that is about to change.

Here is the Personal Health Analysis checklist that I use with my clients. What I'd like you to do is complete this personal health analysis sheet four times a year. That will help you determine just how you're progressing towards your given goals. Get started now! Keep your personal analysis checklist on hand and watch your changes unfold in black and white.

Personal Health Analysis

How many 8 oz servings of the following do you drink each day?
a) Coffee _____ □Regular □Decaf
   What do you put in your coffee?_____
b) Tea _____ □Regular □Herbal
   What do you put in your tea? _____
c) Soda _____ □Regular □Diet
d) Energy/Sports Drinks _____
e) Water _____
f) Alcohol _____
g) Juices _____ What kind?_____

Give a brief description of a typical day of eating for you.
Breakfast:_____
Morning Snack: _____
Lunch: _____
Afternoon Snack:_____
Dinner:_____
Evening Snack: _____

Do you use any artificial sweetener? □Yes □No

How many times a week do you eat fast food?_____
Processed foods?_____

Do you tend to have cravings? ▢Yes ▢No
What do you crave?_____

Do you eat organic foods? ▢Yes ▢No

Are you on any prescription medications? ▢Yes ▢No
What medical condition are they for?_____
_____

Do you have any other medical conditions that you are under a
doctor's care for? ▢Yes ▢No
If yes, what are they?_____

Do you have any allergies? ▢Yes ▢No
If yes, what kind? _____

Have you ever had cancer? ▢Yes ▢No
If yes, what kind?_____
When?_____
Have you ever had radiation or chemotherapy? ▢Yes ▢No

With any of your medical conditions, have you ever been told not to
eat certain foods or vitamins? ▢Yes ▢No

Do you currently smoke? ▢Yes ▢No If yes, how many daily? _____

Have you ever smoked? ▢Yes ▢No
If yes, when did you quit?_____

Are you pregnant or nursing? ▢Yes ▢No

How many bowel movements do you have per day?_____
per week?_____ Ever had bowel problems? ▢Yes ▢No
If yes, what was the problem?_____

Have you ever had stomach problems? □Yes □No
If yes, what was the problem?_____

What other programs/diets have you tried?

_____

Have you tried cleansing before? □Yes □No

What nutritional supplements do you take?

_____

Do you currently exercise? □Yes □No
If No, have you ever exercised before? □Yes □No

What is your highest value in life?_____

_____

On a scale of 1-10 (with 10 being the best):
How would you rate your overall health?_____
Where would you LIKE it to be? _____
How would you rate your overall energy?_____
Where would you LIKE it to be?_____

On a scale of 1-10 (with 10 being the worst):
How would you rate your level of stress?_____
Where would you LIKE it to be?_____

What benefits would you like to experience?
□ Removal of impurities   □ Build lean muscle mass
□ Less discomfort   □ Get rid of a bad habit
□ Improved mobility   □ Better athletic performance
□ Increased energy   □ Improved digestion
□ Enhanced mental clarity   □ Decreased stress levels
□ Better sleep   □ Improve a relationship
□ Sugar balance
□ Other: _____

Is weight loss or gain something you'd like to experience? □Yes □No
If so, how much, in sizes _____ or pounds _____?
What time frame _____?

On a scale of 1-10 (with 10 being the best) how important is it for you
to reach these goals? _____

I am 100 percent committed to your success. What type of support
do you think you will need to reach your goals?
_____

How would you describe your commitment to attain these goals?
□ High   □ Medium   □ Low

 List the positive people in your life who want you to succeed
_____
_____
_____
_____

 Is there anyone you would like to be accountable to?
_____

Weight, measurements, and picture done? □Yes □No

After 90 days . . . Goals accomplished:_____
_____
_____
_____
_____
_____
_____

90 day weight, measurements, and picture done? □Yes □No
If yes, what changes have you seen? _____
_____

Learn How to Eat to Live Instead of Living to Eat

The first step in recovery from any addiction is to recognize and acknowledge that you have that addiction. When I realized that I was a food addict, I knew that I had become the sort of person who lived to eat (sometimes all day long).

How, then, could I completely transform my attitude and eating habits, so that I would be one of those people who ate only when she was hungry and eats to live instead of the other way around?

Here are a few ways that worked for me to turn that mental switch from "on" to "off" when it came to changing my attitude about food.

What's Your "Why?"

The most important step I took in eating better was to decide my "why." Ask yourself why you want to eat healthier, release weight, and transform your life. Is it because you want to be able to play tag with your kids? Climb a mountain with your husband? Fit into your old wedding dress? Do you want to live until you die, instead of dying and then sticking around for a few more years while your kids take care of you?

My own "why" was twofold: I was tired of sitting on the bench at the park and not being one of those moms who plays with her kids, and I wanted to be able to inspire and serve other people. Those two goals kept me going. If I could struggle with my weight throughout my whole life, yet finally achieve the goal of a healthier, leaner body, then others can, too.

Do you love your life enough to change it? If you're reading this book, you already know the answer to that question. Now take the next step and ask yourself why you want to change your life. What do you want to be monumentally different in your life? Whatever your answer, write it down and pin it up on your vision board, then find an image to support it. This "why" will keep inspiring you to live your dream.

Plan Meals Simply, Yet Carefully

It's easier to hide food or binge when you're alone. I have a friend who would buy 100 large chocolate bars at Christmas time and hide them in his gun safe so that he knew he had his "go to" chocolate stash available at all times. Stop hiding food in your car, bookshelf, special cupboard, desk, or nightstand. Be honest with yourself and with others. Get rid of your secret stashes and keep food out in the open. Plan out healthy meals in advance, as I noted earlier in the book, and eat high protein snacks to avoid blood sugar dips and those "I'm so hungry I'm gonna crash if I don't eat now!" scenarios. It's about preparation. The more prepared you are, the smaller the chance of eating something you shouldn't.

It also helps to portion out single servings on smaller plates. Always eat your meals at the dinner table, not in the car or in front of the TV. If your mind is on your food and not on something else, you're more likely to track what you're eating more accurately rather than binging before you've noticed. If you're a mom who tends to finish what's on your kids' plates as you clear the dishes, immediately pour their leftover drinks or water over the food so that it is no longer appetizing.

Eating in a healthier way is all about preparation and planning. Be sure that healthy food is already in your house and know some "go to" healthy dinner recipes. Always eat regularly, too, so that you can keep your blood sugar levels on an even keel. I was taught that a good rule of thumb in keeping your blood sugar stable is to have protein, fat, and complex carbs together. Personally, I avoid gluten, white flour, sugar, dairy, and red meat.

It might take a few months to change your eating patterns. Once you do, you'll get used to eating smaller amounts of food and healthier nutrients that will automatically help squash those fast food and sugar cravings.

In with the Good, Out with the Bad

If you're like me, you'll reach for that bag of Oreos or other sweet treat in your cupboard when you're hungry or stressed. The more you eat sugary foods, the more your taste buds get used to that flavor and the more your brain will crave even sweeter foods. The chemical makeups of many processed foods have addictive properties as well. These addictive flavors make it so that no matter how much you eat, you're never quite satisfied. For instance, I could sit down and eat a bag of chips whether I wanted them or not, but who sits down and eats a bag of apples? So, what does that mean? That means you need to take the things you know are addictive for you, whether they're salty treats or sweet ones, and remove them from your diet.

What can you do to reprogram your taste buds? Stop giving in by "accident." What I mean is that you must start reading labels so that you know what you are really eating. You owe it to yourself to become informed about the food that you're putting into your body. When you buy foods that aren't expected to have sugar, like pasta sauce, bread, and crackers, make sure they don't have additional artificial sweeteners. Sometimes you are better off with the "regular" version of foods because many of the lower-fat or lower-calorie foods are actually higher in sugar. Stay away from processed foods as best you can. The less you have, the less you will crave. Substitute fruits and veggies to restore the sensitivity in your taste buds. Remember that a healthy body craves healthy food, and a sick body craves sick food.

Know Yourself and Your Weaknesses

I love sugar. Other people crave popcorn, peanuts, even alcohol. The important thing is to know your own weaknesses. If you're like me and can't resist that basket of hot rolls that a waitress always brings at your favorite restaurant, tell her not to bring the basket! And, if you can't say no to dessert, ask her to please not bring you the dessert menu. At home, if you know you can't eat just one brownie, either make them and give them all away or don't make them at all. If you can't avoid popping in for a treat every time you drive past your favorite bakery or fast food place, take a different route on your way home from work. And, if it's your own kitchen that's the den of temptations for you, redo your cupboards until you could eat everything in those cupboards without feeling too guilty.

Holidays can prove especially difficult. My best trick for Halloween is to either by something other than candy to give away, or only buy candy that I don't like and purchase it no sooner than the day before. That way, the trick-or-treaters actually get their treats!

It Shouldn't Be All or Nothing

I know how tempting it is to be an "all or nothing" kind of eater, because that's who I was! The minute somebody told me that I couldn't eat a certain food, well, that's the food I craved more than anything on earth, so I gorged on it. That's another sign of an addictive mindset.

The trick to succeeding at dieting is to not diet. That's right. You heard me: don't think of yourself as being on a diet, and don't tell people that you're on a diet. Just think of this as a time in your life when you're choosing to eat better and get healthier. Forget the days of bouncing between overstuffed and sick to feeling starved. Just eat when you're hungry and eat a little less than you want. Think of starving as being zero on a scale and feeling overly full as the number ten on that same scale. Then try to stay at number five. Mindfully stop eating when you're no longer hungry rather than waiting until you're stuffed.

And probably here is the most important rule of all: when you ingest foods that are lacking nutrients, your body and brain are never satisfied. When you feed your body the nutrients it needs, your brain will let you know when it is satisfied.

Deal with Your Issues

If you've written your burn letter, then you can probably see your own food addiction patterns and highlight the emotions linked to your eating patterns. Once you do that, you can deal with the real issues in your life and stop relying on food for comfort. You can then tackle problems head on instead of numbing your emotions with a sweet treat or a salty bag of chips.

Is your job a drag? Are you in a relationship that seems to leave you depressed and worried instead of feeling supported and loved? Do you have friends that take more from you than they give? Once you can identify and manage your emotional low points, you'll find that you won't "need" to eat quite so often for comfort. You need to be honest with yourself first. Second, put yourself in surroundings that support you as much as possible. For some people, this means acknowledging whom you feel good around and whom you don't. Others might need a 12-step program or therapy. The point is to identify the best and most supportive environments for you and then make a conscious habit of surrounding yourself with that support.

Find Healthier Ways to Cope with Life's Ups and Downs

As a food addict, I used to reward myself with food—even when I lost weight! It's easy to substitute food with other addictions that might harm your health, like alcohol or cigarettes. Now I know that I have to replace my food addiction with something more positive. For me, that has turned out to be exercise, since exercise sparks the same pleasure centers in the brain that food does. I know that exercise will help my metabolism keep going at a steady clip. It will also help my mind remain clear and calm and raise the level of my endorphins, those feel-good hormones. You could also try going out with friends who always make you feel upbeat, or see a therapist who can help you replace food with something that will turn out to be even more emotionally fulfilling.

If you're not physically hungry yet have a sudden craving, here are some other things to try: drink water, brush your teeth, leave the house for a minute, or eat a piece of fruit or a handful of vegetables. First and foremost, though, ask yourself why you're experiencing a craving. Take a deep breath or two and give yourself time to pause and reflect on your emotions before you react to them.

Keep a Food and Gratitude Journal

I know that I said this earlier in the book, however it's vitally important and bears repeating: one of the best ways to be accountable for what you eat is to write it down. Buy a journal or a notebook and keep it handy—in your purse or on your nightstand—or use your smartphone. Any way you can do it honestly, record everything you eat and be accurate about the amounts. Write down what you eat, morsel by morsel as well as what you're feeling as you consume that food. Maybe even mention what's going on in your life at the moment, so that you can connect even further to your feelings as they relate to food. Doing so will give you a good insight into your own food addiction patterns and will help you learn to manage them.

One last important thing to record: include 10 things you are grateful for that day. While I know this isn't always easy, I know you can do it! One day I had the stomach flu. I was feeling horrible and, basically, staying in bed all day long. When it came time to write in my gratitude journal, I couldn't think of a single thing to write. Right then and there, I discovered that I was so thankful for my bed that I was lying in, the bowl that was next to me, and my toilet for sure. I also gave thanks that my kids were so good to play by themselves all day long.

Gratitude is the highest form of vibration. It brings you closest to God and also puts out into the universe the positive energy that you deserve in return. A group of friends and I decided to text each other what we were grateful for before we even climbed out of bed each morning. It begins each and every day with the "attitude of gratitude."

Forgive Yourself

Many people give up on releasing weight because they don't succeed right away. That's too bad, because if you learn to forgive yourself immediately when you slip up, then that momentary slip-up won't turn into an entire day, a week, or even a whole year. Keep moving forward toward your goals instead of sliding back.

It's important to know that we all slip up. Although I lost half of my body weight, even now I have to be mindful in order to keep on track. Just recently, I went through a tough emotional time and ended up packing on 15 pounds in record time. You know what? Just like you, I had to forgive myself and say, "Okay, enough." Now I'm refocused and taking good care of myself, so that I can keep living my dream of a healthier, better life.

Slipping up is something everyone does; it's what you do afterward that really matters. For people like us, it's a slippery slope. Abstinence from trigger foods is ideal. If you do slip up, recognize it as quickly as possible, forgive yourself, and get back on track. You will see it happen less and less as you develop more confidence in your own recovery.

Treat Your Body Like the Miracle It Is

Loving yourself means learning to love your body, too—just as it is right now. This isn't always easy, especially if you're feeling flabby and overweight, as I did before my transformation. I used to dislike looking at myself in mirrors so much that I would avoid turning my head in that direction if I walked into a room with one. Or, even worse, I'd stare at myself in the bathroom mirror and weep over the huge image in front of me.

These days, I'm much more aware of the fact that the human body is truly nothing short of a miracle—and definitely something to be appreciated every day. Just think of all the things your body has already allowed you to experience and create! An underused body is an unappreciated body, and you owe it to yourself and to your body to help it do everything it is capable of doing. Think of someone who doesn't have that choice and feel grateful for the choices you *do* have.

Learning to love and appreciate your body begins with cleansing your body of impurities, not just through nutritional cleansing, but by learning to eat cleaner, leaner foods as well as learning to manage the stress you expose yourself to in your environment. You're going to feel better and love your body more if you appreciate where those two legs can take you, how hard that generous heart of yours can pump when you're exercising, and what your hands can do with a ball or a set of weights. Your body is a miracle of a machine. It just needs to be set in motion for you to learn to love it and truly appreciate all that it can do for you.

Cleansing

People have all of these notions about what "cleansing" is. They use this word to describe everything from cleaning out your colon to living on fruit juice all day. What I'm talking about when I say "cleansing" is nutritional cleansing at the cellular level and supporting your liver.

Picture your liver with a front and back door. If your body is working efficiently, both doors are open so that impurities are filtered through the liver and can leave the body. When your body isn't working well, the impurities go in the front door; however, not all of them can leave through the back door. Instead, they stay in your system. You feel tired and your body doesn't work efficiently, not to mention the fact that the impurities that don't get filtered out of your body will, instead, stay in your system.

Your body needs specific nutrients to create a healthy cell. Most of us try to "eat right" because we're aware—even if we don't do it every day—that our bodies need a certain nutritional mix to have the high-powered fuel they need to perform their functions efficiently. However, what I feel most diets and nutritional programs lack is cleansing—not just a specific cleanse that targets one or two organs in your body, but a full-body, nutritional cleanse that cleanses deeper, on a cellular level. When you cleanse out the impurities and feed the body the nutrients it needs, your body begins to function efficiently, as it was designed to.

For me, cleansing was the missing link to the weight loss and wellness puzzle. If I had known about cleansing clear back in third grade, I wouldn't have struggled with weight my whole life. I feel that with the proper nutritional program, cleansing will help flush the impurities out of your body as you stay healthy and release weight, keep the weight off, and maintain your lean muscle tissue at the same time.

Eating Clean

Many, many people ask me what the best nutritional approach is for optimal health. Should we be eating low carb foods? Low sugar? No dairy or meat? Only meat and veggies? Or what?

These are great questions because there is no one perfect way to eat. You have to look at your own unique body chemistry and personal nutrition goals. It's about being in tune to and listening to your body.

It is worth looking at the government's new MyPlate guidelines, which have replaced the Food Pyramid, for a basic understanding of what experts consider to be optimal nutrition. Those guidelines say that each meal should be a small dinner plate where half the dinner plate is fruits and veggies (with 2/3 more veggies than fruit), and the other half is divided between complex carbohydrates and a serving of lean protein.

In other words, the nutrition experts all agree that low glycemic foods that include healthy carbs is the clean way of eating that we all should be following. (If you have young kids, you can actually buy dinner plates that have sections built in to teach them portions and food groups. They're great!) So, when I say "healthy carbs," I'm not saying "no carbs." I'm just asking you to eat healthy complex carbs, keeping the glycemic index in mind. You can find the glycemic index all over the Internet. Basically, the lower the number in the index, the less your blood sugar spikes when you eat it. The more even your blood sugar level stays, the more efficient your body works.

That said, let me tell you what I did. In my view, the most nutritionally disruptive foods that everyone should cut from their diets are soda, coffee, white flour, and white sugar. It's also a good idea to limit dairy, pork and red meat. Though I didn't go off red meat completely, I did go off the others. Not only were some of these trigger foods for me, I feel they were also inflammatory, keeping my body in a state of constant turmoil as my cells fought the inflammation instead of calmly allowing good nutrients to assimilate in my body.

I never stopped eating fruit; I still eat one piece of fruit per day. To make sure that I don't feel hungry, and, to counteract the sugar spike you get from fruit, I always combined my fruit with a protein like raw almonds or a tablespoon of organic peanut or almond butter. In fact, my favorite treat, which I save for early afternoon if I get the munchies, is an apple and peanut butter.

When it comes to fruits and veggies, make it a point to eat as raw as possible. By this, I mean that you should try to get most of your daily nutrition from uncooked, unprocessed foods. Know where your foods come from, too; for instance, you want to make sure that you choose a lean source of protein like chicken, turkey, fish, or legumes. Ideally, these should be organic, wild, or free-range protein sources, without hormones or antibiotics. If you do choose to eat beef or dairy, choose grass-fed and hormone- and antibiotic-free—always the healthiest option. It's important to know the quality of the food you put into your body and where it comes from.

For the rest of your calories, consider these options:

Vegetables

Veggies (prepared raw, steamed, broiled, or grilled), up to 24 ounces of vegetables a day, spread out between snacks and lunch or in one sitting. Be creative and try something new!

Healthy Fats

About 2 tablespoons of healthy fat every day like olive, coconut or walnut oils, avocados, green olives, or nuts. If you opt for salad dressing, don't use low fat; these tend to have extra sugar. It's better to use a small amount of the real thing.

Salads

I like a salad most every day. I will add a cooked turkey burger and have it with tomatoes, garlic, and yummy seasonings. Maybe add black beans—I really enjoy my salad that way! Some people say that salads don't fill them up. It's because they need to add protein. Protein takes longer to digest and lets you feel full longer.

Grains

A nutritional counselor told me that taking grains out of my diet in the beginning was good for my pancreas and would help aid my weight loss. So if you want to go all-out like I did, go off your grains for the first 30 days or longer if you are able and then add them back in very slowly if you choose to. This includes whole wheat bread, pastas, and even brown rice. I feel this to be especially important if you have over 100 pounds to release, as I did. When adding them back into your diet, pay attention to how you feel. Do you feel bloated? Are you finding that you crave them? If that were the case, I would remove them completely.

A Few Quick Recipes

Shrimp with Marinara Sauce and Steamed Broccoli: Boil or grill the shrimp. Top it with a low-sugar marinara (We use our homemade marinara; we usually do a very large batch at once and then use it as we need.) and put just ½ ounce of Romano cheese on it. Delicious.

"Spaghetti": Make with spaghetti squash and a low-sugar marinara sauce; serve with grilled chicken, shrimp, or salmon.

Turkey Burgers: 2 ½ lbs. of ground turkey made with 2 finely-diced onions, ¼ red and ¼ green peppers, add in 2 packages of taco seasoning, a few dashes of Worcestershire sauce, and 2 eggs. Mix all ingredients together, weigh out into individual portion sizes, grill, and freeze extras. It makes 10 servings and is SO GOOD! You could also make this into a meatloaf and cut it into 10 servings.

Tuna, Turkey, or Chicken Lettuce Wraps, No Cheese: Use lettuce leaves instead of bread, roll up, and enjoy!

Chicken Stir-Fry: My grocery store actually has a frozen bean mixture—white, yellow, and green beans with carrots. Measure out individual servings of cooked chicken in containers and set it aside. Next, sauté some onions and the frozen bean mixture in a few servings of olive oil, add in some eggplant, season it, measure out ½ cup servings, and then add it to the cooked chicken. This is great to freeze for later!

White Chili: We use lentils, celery, onions, carrots, and green chilies (We use the mild ones for our kids.) and cook them in a Crock-Pot until they are tender. You can add chicken. The chilies really add a lot of flavor. Then add just a small amount of yogurt to give it the creaminess you are expecting.

Black Bean Soup: Just black beans, onions, carrots, celery, seasonings—it's awesome! Sometimes I add salsa to give it an extra kick.

Black Bean Fajitas: Black beans cooked with shredded zucchini, onions, and fajita seasoning. YUMMY!

No-Crust Quiche/Frittata: Use eggs and egg beaters together, a little water for the fluffy egg/omelet effect, and then fill it with veggies—sautéed peppers, broccoli, onions, and fresh tomatoes. We serve it with salsa. I sometimes add just ½ ounce of cheese to the top of each serving.

Tuna Boats: Believe it or not, my kids love these! We get romaine lettuce leaves and make up tuna salad with just tuna and a tiny bit of mayonnaise. Then we fill the "boats" with it and serve. I'll make tuna boats for me and tuna melts for the kids and they usually ask for mine! Add a slice of avocado to that and you have a special treat!

Oatmeal Pancakes: Mix five egg whites with one whole egg. Add ¼ cup oatmeal and mix. Cook it in a skillet as one big pancake. Transfer to a plate, top with salsa and guacamole. So yummy!

Dining Out

If you are going to a restaurant, check the menu out online first. Look for the healthiest options so that you know what you will be ordering before you get there. Don't be afraid to ask for modifications. Remember that you are paying for service and your server wants you to have what is right for you. They will be happy to accommodate you. Ask for things like dressing on the side and ask to replace the starch in the entrée with an extra serving of the veggies. Ask how things are prepared. Are the vegetables sautéed? Ask for them grilled or steamed. Is there a sauce for the entrée? Ask for it on the side. Just because you're changing how you eat doesn't mean you can't eat out!

Get Off the Couch!

If you're like I once was, you don't know the value of exercise. Maybe you don't want to walk around your neighborhood because you feel self-conscious about the way people look at you, or you're so out of breath just getting the newspaper out of the mailbox that you can't imagine walking from your house to the corner.

Here's the truth, which I had to discover the hard way: it's never too late to get your body moving—and there is never a more important moment to start exercising than right now, when you're determined to transform your body and your life. Exercise won't just help you release weight; it will help lift your mood, give you energy, and provide mental clarity, especially if you head outdoors and connect with nature.

If you're too self-conscious to walk where people can see you, find a quieter street or a neighborhood where nobody knows you. I always say that what people think of *you* is none of *your* business!

Or, if exercising outdoors poses too much of challenge at first, walk in place and do leg lifts and push-ups in the comfort of your own house. You can get an exercise DVD or just put on your favorite music. See if your television service offers an exercise channel or on-demand exercise videos. If you don't have that option, go to your local library and see if they offer videos to check out.

If videos are too much for you in the beginning, begin slowly. Start on the edge of the kitchen counter, pushing with your arms in a mini-push-up as you begin, or lie on your side and lift your leg while you watch TV instead of just sitting. Stand on the edge of a step and do calf raises or lunges and squats while you are doing things around the house. Resistance exercises like these build your lean muscle tissue over time, which in turn will burn more calories, assisting you in keeping your weight off. Resistance (weight training) exercises can also help reshape your body. Anything is better than nothing. The more you move, the more you'll want to. You'll find that your body feels better when you move around. Our bodies are meant to be used.

See your doctor for a physical before you begin doing any exercise if it has been a long while since you moved around. Once your health care practitioner gives you a thumbs-up, start with 15 to 30 minutes of gentle cardio every other day, depending on how well you tolerate exercise, and gradually work up to an hour. That can be as simple as walking 15 minutes in one direction, turning around and walking back. To be sure you are getting the cardio benefits, you should be able to carry on a conversation feeling a little out of breath.

Once you get a handle on cardio exercises, consider trying

interval training. That is my favorite cardio to do. I sweat and burn so many more calories in a shorter period of time.

I've listed some gentle, easy exercises here that you can do right at home on the days you aren't doing your cardio. These exercises will build your core muscles:

(3) reps of 5–15 "press-ups" (lay on your belly on the ground and just press up with your arms in push-up position)

(3) reps of 5–15 "press-ups with hands closer together"

(3) reps of 5–15 "regular push-ups" (you can start on your knees and work up to on your toes)

(3) reps of 15 counts of planks (on elbows)

(3) reps of 15 counts of side planks (right & left)

(3) reps of 15 lunges (right & left) or do walking lunges

(3) reps of squats and (3) reps of leg lifts (right & left)

(3) reps of 15 abdominal crunches

Again, these are suggestions just to get you started. Google these exercises to find videos to show proper form. You will find that, once you start searching, there are many others. These particular exercises use several muscles at once, keeping your workout time efficient as well as effective.

What's most important is finding a type of exercise that you enjoy. Maybe you're someone who needs to work out with someone. If so, find a walking partner. If you're someone that likes to do something different every day, find some programs online that you can do at home. Whatever you choose, schedule it like an appointment for yourself and try to do it consistently. Start with three days per week and go from there. The goal is to make exercise something that is part of your life on a regular basis as well as something you can reasonably do. So be sure the time you schedule is appropriate, particularly in the beginning.

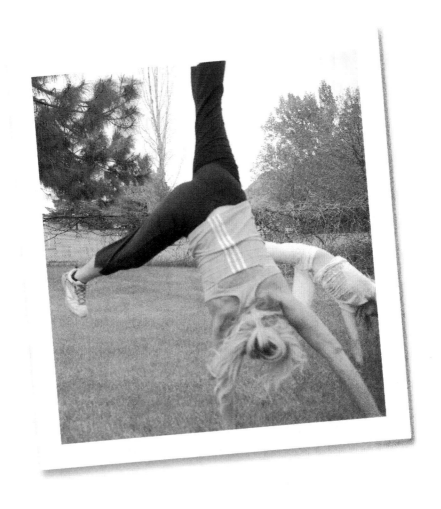

12

REMEMBER WHERE IT CAME FROM

*Only you can make yourself truly happy
and live like the new you.*

— Jill Birth

As you begin releasing weight and transforming your body, watch how it resonates with many of the things on your vision board. This is because you will become more confident and creative in listening to your own inner voice instead of believing the things other people may have believed about you. You will find your voice and use it—especially if it means making your wishes heard. As you learn to ask for what you want, you will begin to receive it. Your mindfulness and newfound belief in yourself will help you realize things on your vision board. You will be amazed.

Where does a dream go after you've dreamed it? That's a great question! While it will be a wonderful transition as you begin controlling what you eat, releasing weight, moving around more, and living your dream, it may not necessarily be an easy one. You may have to deal with many conflicting emotions as you shed your old life and begin this new, exciting one and live your dream. Just be mindful that this discomfort indicates change, and *change is good*.

For instance, many of us are fortunate to have wonderful support on this journey of transformation. I had my friends, family, and coworkers all cheering me on. However, you may discover—as I did—that some relationships alter as people react to the trimmer, fitter, and more confident you. There was one particularly painful incident in my life, for example. This involved a close girlfriend, one with whom I had always shared birthday celebrations—usually a nice lunch to mark my special day or hers. Not long after I won the Transformation Challenge, I telephoned this friend near her birthday to arrange lunch. And, you know what? She refused to go out with me. She said she was no longer interested in being my friend because I wasn't the same person!

In a way, she was right. Physically and mentally I wasn't the same—in a good way. I was happier than ever, yet still the same Jill. I didn't understand why she couldn't be happy for me. I was disheartened and confused. I knew people who had improved their lives and I was happy for them. Had I confused friendship with being the safe, fat friend?

Many other people also treated me so differently that it made my head spin. Men who never would have given me a second glance paid attention to me now that I was a thin, athletic-looking blonde. People in my own neighborhood—the women, especially—made catty remarks about my appearance and the money I had won. A few of the girls in the office wouldn't even turn around and say hello when I came into work. And my marriage, which I kept hoping for so many years might improve, continued to slide downward, despite the fact that I now looked pretty much like the wife I thought Dave had wanted all along. We were no closer emotionally than we had been before.

So I was still sad and confused, sometimes, despite my new look. Since I am the kind of person who loves everyone, it was really hard for me to accept the idea that some people weren't going to like me anymore because of the way I looked now—just as some people didn't like me when I was obese because they were ashamed to be seen with me. It took a lot of counseling for me to learn that people who behave like this do so out of their own insecurities and issues. That was truly an uphill battle for me. It still is, sometimes. The people I love are loved for who they are on the inside, not what they look like on the outside. So, needless to say, I wasn't prepared for some of these reactions. Now I try to remember that they were the minority. The rest were happy for me, which I very much appreciated.

While our insecurities can cause us to worry that we're not good enough or that maybe we need to appear less happy, resist. Pray for the people who make you feel that way, knowing that their own insecurities are the reason they're behaving like this. This is their backpack full of stones, not yours.

I'm saying all of this to you because I want you to remember where you have come from as you move on to a new place. Take that love letter to yourself and put it someplace where you can see it regularly to remind yourself of all of the goodness you have inside you—no matter how quickly or slowly you transform on the outside, or how people treat you. What other people think of you doesn't matter nearly as much as what you think of yourself. It's not about ego. It's about love.

How do you continue loving yourself as you struggle to get to and then maintain your perfect weight and live your dreams? Here are a few tips to help you protect your confidence and guide you on your way.

Remember Your "Why"

Why did you choose to become healthier and change your life? Here is an exercise that can help you understand and stay focused on your goal. On a clean sheet of paper, draw a circle and write in the center of it your biggest "Why" for wanting to transform your body and your life. Then draw an arrow from the left to the "Why" in the

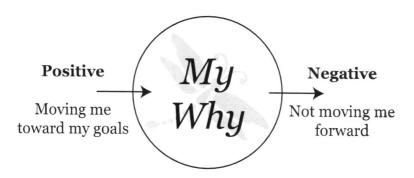

Positive — Moving me toward my goals

My Why

Negative — Not moving me forward

center and another from the "Why" going out to the right.

On the right hand side of the page, make a list of every negative thought, every bit of drama, every phone call you are holding onto, and every negative thing that is not productive or not moving you forward. Those things are taking away from your "Why." See if those things are more important than what you wrote in your circle. And if they aren't, let them go. The goal is for the left side of your "Why" to be happily unbalanced.

On the left side of the page, list everything that is helping you take care of and achieve your "Why." Each day, choose how much time you are going to spend on each side—those things adding to and those things taking away from your "Why."

This exercise will help you stay focused on putting energy into the positive side of your life's equation!

Never Compare Yourself to Others

No matter what shape you're in, how much you weigh, who loves you, or what you're doing with your life, you will always be able to find some people who are worse off than you are and some people who are doing better. There is no reason to compare yourself to anyone. The only things you should keep in mind are your own goals and your own progress towards those goals—one step at a time. Those are the only things you can keep in check.

Remember that you're winning even if you fall off the wagon

and fail now and then. Desiring your goal enough to get up and move towards it tomorrow, no matter what happened today, means that you're learning something new about yourself every day. You gain strength, courage, and confidence from every experience that makes you stop, look fear in the face, and do the very thing you think you cannot do.

Be Grateful for Who You Are

Focusing on your weaknesses is a sure path to failure and despair. Instead, concentrate on your own gifts and strengths. Remember to write down 10 things you're grateful for every day and read them over. Don't envy what others are doing. Focus on your own natural talents and gifts and work those! Think of the things that you know you do well and surround yourself with people who appreciate those gifts and can help you grow even stronger. Find other people who are strong where you are weak, so that they can teach you how to overcome your own weaknesses. Surround yourself with grateful people and positive energy as often as possible. Focus on what you have and what you're grateful for.

Accept What Comes and See the Positive

Success happens in different ways and at different times for everybody. You have to be ready to accept what comes to you. You have to give yourself permission to be more than what you are right now. You were put on this earth to thrive and have a prosperous life and to help others, too. Allow yourself to have it and enjoy it. You deserve it.

My kids and I play a game that we call, "What's great about this?" One Christmas Eve, I was running around trying to get last minute things done before a party I was giving at my house that night. My two youngest children were ages two and four. I went shopping for some last minute items, and when I left the store to go to the car, I realized that I had locked my keys in the car. I wanted to cry. Instead, I took a deep breath, went back into the store, finally found a locksmith that would come on Christmas Eve, put my kids back in the cart, and went to the toy department. We went and looked at every toy in the whole store while waiting for the locksmith.

My kids were so happy that I stopped rushing and spent quality time with them. We sang Christmas songs all the way home. So, when something happens, good or bad, stop and thank God for your blessings, and say, *"What's great about this?"* Sometimes it may be hard. I know you'll learn a lesson in every situation. When you break a glass bottle on the floor, at least every speck of the floor gets clean, right? See the positive or at least the lesson in the situation. After all, learning from a situation is a positive step forward.

When You're Down, Lift Yourself Up by Serving Others

Many negative thoughts stem from fear. When you're having a less-than-stellar day, push the negative thoughts away. Nothing conquers fear faster than faith and taking action. Pick something on your vision board and make a move toward it. Have a list of simple, daily actions handy, too, so that you can pull them out and pick an activity when you're feeling blue or discouraged: walk the dog, pull weeds from the garden, write a thank you note to somebody who has helped you, clean out that hall closet, or help a friend. Any activity that makes you feel productive and better about yourself can go on that list!

No activity will make you feel better than serving others. I feel service is the best way to distract yourself and be blessed at the same time. We become so caught up in the business of our lives. If we just step back and take a good look at what we're doing, we may find that we have immersed ourselves in the "thick of thin things." In other words, too often we spend most of our time taking care of things that don't really matter much at all in the grand scheme of life, while neglecting those more important causes.

When I was focusing every day on what I was going to eat

next, obsessing over what diet I was going to try or how much I was going to weigh the next day, I was only thinking about myself and not others. When we aren't living in our best bodies, we tend to dwell on ourselves, and therefore, aren't in a place to be of service.

I love the scripture that says: *Do unto others, as you would have them do unto you* (Luke 6:31). Make that your motto to live by and it will be easy to lift your spirits when you're down.

Be Where You Are

Nobody is perfect. Your life will still be full of mountains to climb as well as unexpected potholes in the road. A perfect life would be a boring life!

Instead, be willing to take risks even though you may fail. Do what you can with what you have, and there you are! Savor the journey as you learn more about yourself and the world each day. Everyone who has ever reached any kind of success has felt inadequate and embarrassed and wanted to quit at some point on their journeys. Most of the important things in the world have been accomplished by people who have kept on trying when there seemed to be no help at all. The people who succeed are the ones who always pick themselves up, learn from the past, and keep going.

We learn to be resilient only by failing, accepting our failures, and trying again. Remember, your journey should be about your progress, not about being perfect! You are worthy of getting up and moving forward. Just remember to learn something from the process along the way. You grow when you learn from your missteps. You deserve to keep growing.

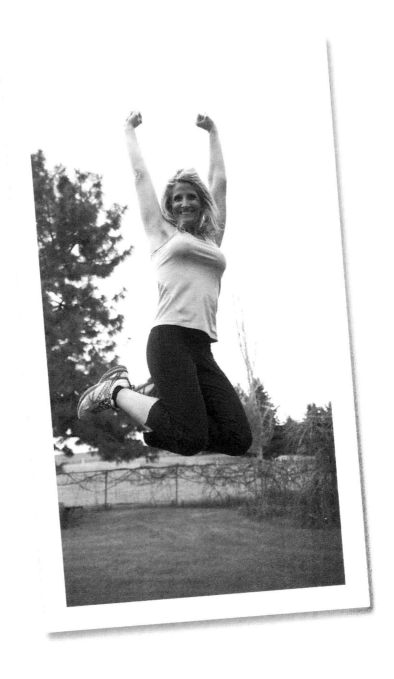

13

NEVER STOP DREAMING

Have the courage to be the person you always wanted to be, the person God *intends* for you to be.

— Jill Birth

Living your dream won't always be easy. It's a daily effort to be our best selves whether we're struggling to improve our fitness, release weight, advance our careers, be closer to the people we love, or love ourselves. Even when you reach the goals you set for yourself, there will be more waiting for you—a way to set the bar higher as you continue to live your dream, and dream your future.

It has been a year and a half since I won the Transformation Challenge. I released an incredible 131 pounds—half my body weight! I have gone from a size 22 to a size 4. My son and I climbed a mountain together and I ran two half-marathons. I never thought these things would be possible.

You would think that would be enough, right?

It isn't. I still deserve more. You do, too. Because we're human, we must all continue pushing ourselves to accomplish more each day—even if accomplishing "more" means just struggling to stay where we are. Nothing is static. Not our jobs, relationships, or bodies. There will always be more challenges ahead. Emotionally, we have to constantly remind ourselves of our self-worth, telling ourselves that we truly are wonderful, deserving children of God. That happiness is something we all deserve and it begins with gratitude.

I know that I will never again sit on the sidelines when my children are playing. I will go down slides with them, run races, push swings, ride bikes, and even go swimming—something I never thought I'd do—for as long as they'll let me tag along. That was one of my biggest goals, and I've accomplished it. No one can take that away from me, just as nobody can take away your accomplishments.

Remember what First Lady Eleanor Roosevelt once said, "No one can make you feel inferior without your consent." We are worthy of all of it. I belong right there riding bikes with my kids, running races, and going down slides. I not only plan to embrace it all, now I want so much more. I even went skydiving with my son for his 19th birthday!

However, I'm still subject to emotional ups and downs, and those emotional ups and downs sometimes compromise my eating habits if I let them, despite my best efforts. Recently, for instance, my marriage was failing. Ending my marriage was enough to send me into a tailspin that caused me to edge back up the scale by 15 pounds.

What did I do then? You've got it: I renewed my resolve and took them off again! I am human, just like you, and we will never be perfect. We can let tough times allow those negative voices to come back and rent space in our heads. We can allow them to tell us we are failures, that we are unworthy, or . . . we can see that the tough situation is stressful, and, instead of going to the comfort foods and the damaging thoughts we used to indulge in, we can separate ourselves from the situation, choose healthy foods only because we are hungry, protect our recovery, and remind ourselves to see what God sees in us. Remember that vision without action is only a daydream, and action without vision is a nightmare. We must stay focused on our positive vision, including using our vision boards and affirmations, forcing ourselves to add to them and put ourselves in a positive place again.

How did I do it? My husband wanted to stay in our house, so I hunted for a condo I could afford. I kept questioning the Lord, asking Him—and myself—if this was really what I should do. I said, "Okay, Heavenly Father, if this is what I'm supposed to do and what You want for me, I need Your help. I need to find a new condo with great energy. I want a place where my kids can be happy."

As always, I was specific in my wishes. I wanted my condo to be brown, with a rock facing—something very different from where I lived before, for sure! I also asked that my condo be an end unit. Shortly after that, I went on a web site and found a condo three miles away from my current home that had been up for rent for only a few minutes. It was exactly as I had envisioned it!

I phoned the man who owned the condo and told him that I was flying back to Utah from Seattle that night. "I need to see that condo," I said.

"If you're really that serious, I can meet you there tonight," he said.

I flew into Salt Lake City and drove directly to the condo to meet him there. My new home had everything I had asked for! I signed the lease right away.

Once again, opening myself to the universe and being specific in my requests to the Lord had shown me the next, best, significant, life-changing step in my life. I was confident, mindful, focused, and willing to ask God for what I really wanted. God has truly blessed me. I know for sure that God is always looking out for me. God is so good all of the time!

*

Since transforming my own body, I plan to continue doing all I can to help others and pay forward my own good fortune. I want to help people feel as good as I feel today. On a smaller scale, it's not much different than finding a new hairdresser or lipstick you like, or a new gym, and telling people all about this wonderful new thing you've found. I love the thrill of knowing people's lives are improving because of something I may have said or done, because they know that someone cares about them. I see myself as an ambassador of health, and hope to inspire other people to never stop dreaming even after they think they've accomplished everything they thought possible.

Do you want to release 30 pounds? Do you need money to pay for your child's college tuition? Do you want to help your favorite charity? Dream without an agenda. Dream big, and watch what happens.

For my part, I'm still making new goals all of the time. The 12-step program helped me understand what keeps me on track. When I'd reached my goal of running a half-marathon, I realized right away that I needed another physical goal to keep me motivated. I signed up for another race where you run through mud and over obstacles; training for that was fun and kept me focused on fitness in a way that will help me increase my lean muscle mass and lower my percentage of body fat. Always look for new ways to get there.

More importantly, though, the impact of winning the Transformation Challenge and helping other people meet their goals is that I have realized I can accomplish anything I set my mind to—and so can you. It feels fantastic! I want you to have that same incredible feeling! It's a rush. You'll learn that you can have what you choose and live your dream life, and you can help others have it, too.

We need to fill our boxes with all of the talents and abilities God has given us and go and share it with others. Being a positive witness to a healthy, happy life draws people to you, and you feel so good that your confidence to share that feeling is limitless. Imagine saying or doing something that helps someone see things differently, that helps people realize their worth, that gives them the hope and confidence to try once more to change their lives for the better. Remember that your character is your destiny, and often the smallest actions are the ones that have the greatest impact. Think about how powerful and beautiful it is to affect someone's life in a positive way. I get so excited just thinking about it!

My weight is still down and my business has increased tenfold.

I travel and meet lots of people like you, and I love it. I even enjoy public speaking!

At home, my three children now have a mother who has the self-knowledge, confidence, and financial independence to be a good role model for how they might conduct their own lives. Together, we enjoy the fresh air by swimming or hiking and there is always lots to laugh about. It is a life filled with love and hope. The best part is having the peace of mind that I now know how to teach them to live their dreams, which is what all parents want for their children.

Do you know what? For all that I've accomplished, I am just like you. I once felt like a failure. I constantly look to my higher power for guidance. I place my life in God's hands each and every day, realizing that everything happens in His time. You don't need any special magic to live your dream.

Know and believe that you're worthy, start making goals, *find the voice inside you*, and enjoy the journey as you transform your body and your life, one sweet step at a time. Remember your new definition of winning. Your truest self, your courage, and energy for grander dreams, will be boundless. The rewards are endless.

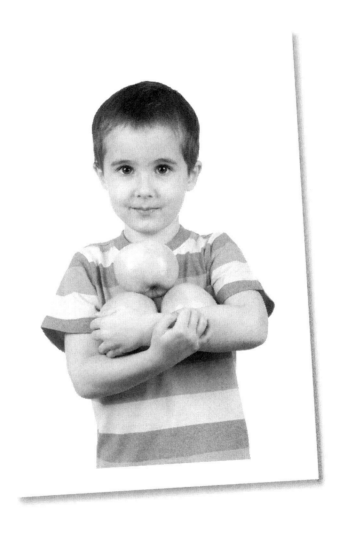

EPILOGUE

PAYING IT FORWARD

Be the change you want to see in the world.

—Mahatma Ghandi

As a child, I used to love watching the dragonflies flit about our cherry orchard when I was hard at work harvesting fruit. I would even rush to save these neon-colored, winged beings from drowning if they fell in the water so they wouldn't die!

What always struck me about these colorful little guys is that they looked so dreamlike, yet prehistoric. Maybe that's because they are: dragonflies were around over 300 million years ago, long before the dinosaurs. Today, scientists have counted about 3000 different dragonfly species around the world, making the dragonfly one of our planet's best examples of evolutionary success.

In many countries around the world, people use the dragonfly as a symbol of change in the process of self-realization—the kind of change that comes from maturing mentally and emotionally as we grapple to understand life's deeper meanings. A dragonfly's iridescent colors change depending on the light; that magical property makes me think about how we discover our own abilities in different situations, by unmasking our real selves and removing our doubts, usually learning we are stronger and have more gifts than we realized.

The fact that dragonflies live only for a few months as adults also reminds me how important it is to live in the moment. That means being aware of who we are, where we are, what we deserve, and what we're doing so that we can make the most informed life choices possible. While we all have to make time to plan, we still need to live each day one day at a time.

Ever since my childhood, I have viewed the dragonfly as a symbol of incredible light, agility, truth, and strength. Today, the dragonfly is a reminder to let my own light shine in the hope that I might inspire you to find your individual light and strength as you transform your body and your life.

As you do, it's important to pay forward your success along the way. That means bringing your family—especially your children—with you on this journey to good health and fitness. This is an important task not just for you, it's important for our country. According to the Centers for Disease Control and Prevention, childhood obesity has more than tripled in the past 30 years, with the percentage of obese children between the ages of 6 and 11 years old increasing from 7 percent in 1980 to nearly 20 percent in 2008. The percentage of obese teens has also increased dramatically, from 5 percent to 18 percent within the same time period. As I discovered in my own life, becoming obese as a child can permanently impact your life and health in a number of harmful ways. I was too self-conscious to speak in my classes or go swimming with friends. I was never asked to a prom and I didn't have a serious relationship until college. I doubted myself as a wife, as a mother, and as a woman.

My childhood obesity left me vulnerable to criticism both from my closest friends and from total strangers. What's more, my lack of self-esteem made it nearly impossible for me to commit to a diet and release weight as an adult, because I already felt like a failure. I didn't believe in myself early in my childhood.

Unfortunately, statistics remind us that my story is far from unique. Obese kids suffer teasing, bullying, and isolation. So many overweight children joke and try to be the "funny friends" in the hopes that people won't see them as obese, when all the while their self-esteem is diminishing more and more. Their emotional problems may lead to deeper body image issues and eating disorders.

Their health suffers also. Obese children are more likely to have risk factors for heart disease—such as high blood pressure or high cholesterol—and are far more likely to have prediabetes, a condition where blood glucose levels indicate that they will develop Type 2 diabetes later. In addition, they're at a greater risk for sleep apnea and bone and joint problems.

What can you do? As you begin your own journey toward a healthier lifestyle, reach back with one hand and bring your children and others in your family with you. You can't just tell your children to eat right and exercise. It's up to you to be the best possible model of behavior for them. Children rarely do what we say. But will usually do what we do. They will joyfully join into a family's team effort, especially if you start while they're young. I've listed a few easy suggestions here for you to try.

Keep the Focus on Eating Healthy Foods, Not on Being Thin

If you're using nutritional products or doing a cleanse, it's far more important to put the focus on being healthy and living a long life than on the weight. The released weight is actually the byproduct of your healthier lifestyle. Frequently explain why something is healthy for them. Use the grocery store as your classroom. Children understand more than you think they do. Talk openly about what foods are nutritious and why our bodies need that kind of fuel.

Regarding my choice to use my nutrient-dense protein shakes and cleansing, I told my children that it was like taking lint out of the dryer so it would work better, I just needed to get clean: "Remember how important it is to clean the lint filter and get all of the bad stuff out? That's what I'm doing."

When I said that, my kids said, "We want to do that, too!" Now I give them a healthy protein shake every morning just to make sure they start the day off right. Now they see that they feel better physically and mentally when they put good nutrition in their bodies, and the days of cold cereal and waffles for breakfast are virtually gone. Given the option, they ask for that shake!

Now, don't get me wrong, we have treats now and then, but they're just that—treats. I don't want my children to think that they can never have them. We just focus on what's healthy and never use food to manage emotions.

Remove Temptation

Sure, you want to clean out those cupboards to remove your own temptations. It's much easier to stick to eating healthy if you can't just grab a bag of chips, so take out the temptations for kids, too. Replace sugary cereals with more low-sugar, higher-fiber, nutrient-dense brands and processed snacks with natural ones. No more potato chips and dip—just whole grain tortilla chips with salsa. Eliminate soda pop and packaged meals like macaroni and cheese, too. Stick with whole wheat pastas, organic fruits, and veggies. Find healthy recipes and have your children get involved in food preparation. Talk about steaming or grilling fresh vegetables as opposed to using canned vegetables or cooking with butter. Broil, grill, and bake your meat, fish, and poultry instead of frying them. It's never too early—or too late—to substitute healthy habits for unhealthy ones.

Make Family Fitness and Fun a Priority

Lots of parents tell their children to exercise because it's "good for you." Here, as in all other situations, children are more apt to follow your lead than your lectures. If you lie around at the beach instead of jumping in the waves, you can expect them to do the same, so get out and get moving as a family. During the summer, I swim, bike, and hike with my kids—even if we just walk a couple of miles every day on the track next to my house. The more fun you have with your children, the less they'll see this as exercise and the more fun these outings will be for all of you. Doing this can instill a love of exercise and the outdoors in your children—the gift of a lifetime. Give them memories they can treasure and habits they can instill in their own children.

Never Reward with Sweet Treats

How many times have you seen another parent distract a weeping child with the promise of a sweet treat, like a lollipop or an ice cream? I've done it in the past. Now I cringe. One of the reasons that our nation is increasingly addicted to food is because we're taught from infancy that food provides comfort.

Use other means to comfort your angry, hurt, or sad child: a hug or eye-to-eye contact at their level, promise them one-on-one time or a favorite story, etc. Think of time and attention as rewards, because those are the most valuable things a parent can give and, deep down, what children need and want most.

If you must use food as a distraction or bribe, choose a healthy snack like a piece of fruit or a whole grain cracker. One of the teachers at our high school made a deal that if his students didn't eat sugar for a whole school year, he would give them each $100. There were many who took on the challenge; eight students succeeded. I'm not saying that this is for everyone. Just try to find an alternative to using food as a reward.

On the other hand, while it is extremely important for us to feed our children nutritious foods and model a healthy, fit lifestyle for them, if your child does have a treat now and then, it should be a pleasurable experience—never a source of guilt. You don't ever want to make your child feel bad about herself over what she eats; rather, send the message that you will love her unconditionally.

Involve Your Kids in Food Preparation

The sooner you involve your children in cooking and packing their own snacks and school lunches, the more they'll understand about nutrition—and the more invested they'll be in assisting to purchase and make healthy meals. Make time to teach them to cook healthy foods. For example, a fun thing to start with is pizza made with whole wheat dough and healthy toppings. Even very young children can help cut up yummy fruit or make a salad and put it in a big bowl.

My own children love packing healthy school lunches, and they're always eager to try something new for dinner—we just bought artichokes to cook for the first time, and we all loved them! The more you can treat healthy eating as an adventure rather than an eat-your-vegetables kind of punishment, the more likely you are to succeed in laying the groundwork for your children to become healthy adults.

If I had my wish, no child would ever have to endure what I did. Children who feel good about their bodies become more confident adults. They end up making healthier decisions all of their now long adult lives if you begin these small changes in your home.

*

In this book, my goal was to help you map out your own success story. I wanted to guide you as you create your own "before" and "after" pictures, while understanding and putting your past behind you, learning to manage your food addiction, and imagining a new vision for your own future—and for your family's future, too. As you find the courage to live your dreams, you will find your truest self.

I know that you will add your unique experiences and voice to help all of our children lead healthier lives. Thank you for letting me share in your wonderful journey. I would love to know how you have taken steps to transform your own life. Stay in touch!

Resources:

To follow my blog and learn about the program that I followed, go to www.jillbirth.com.

I am on Facebook: www.facebook.com/JillsWay

Follow me on Twitter: @jillbirth

To learn more about the LDS 12-step program that I followed go to: http://addictionrecovery.lds.org/struggling-with-addiction?lang=eng

Suggested Reading:

Canfield, Jack and Mark Victor Hansen. *The Aladdin Factor*. New York: Berkeley, 1995.

Canfield, Jack and Jane Switzer. *The Success Principles: How to Get from Where You Are to Where You Want to Be*. New York: Harper Collins, 2005.

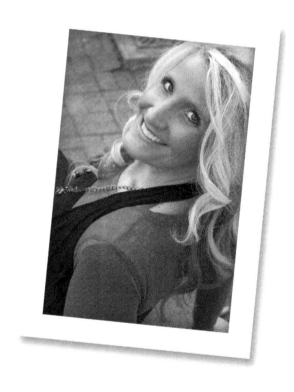

ABOUT THE AUTHOR

Author Jill Birth is a *day maker*—someone whose mission it is to make your day, every day, by helping you finally be done with the weight issues that have been holding you back and by helping you to live the life of your dreams *now*! The mother of three amazing children and a mentor to thousands of people who've successfully found the voices within themselves and transformed their lives, Jill brings her message of hope around the world through motivational speaking. Jill is particularly passionate about ending childhood obesity and is doing what she can to keep the conversation going through education and awareness. Learn more about Jill and her work at www.jillbirth.com.

Our intention creates our reality.

— Wayne Dyer

MY 24 BEFORE PICTURES

They're all here. My favorite? All of them. Why? They're part of my journey—the journey that led me to the 25th picture! While you may see the first 23 as failed attempts, I see them as faith that He would not let me fail.

So feel free to look through the following pages, but be sure to go all the way to the end. That picture is the next phase of my journey—living the life of my dreams!

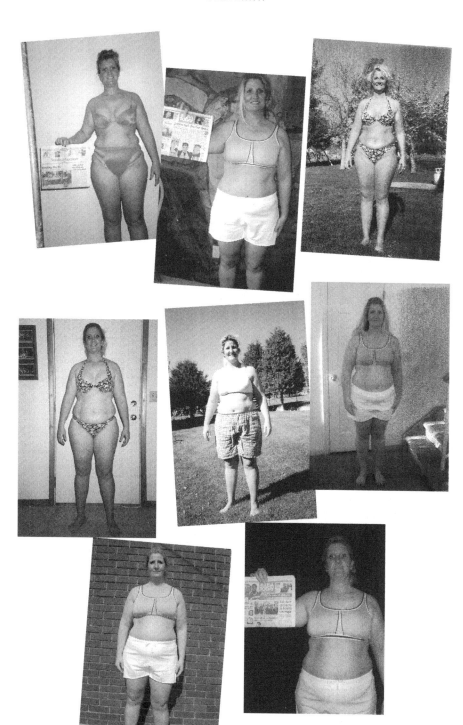

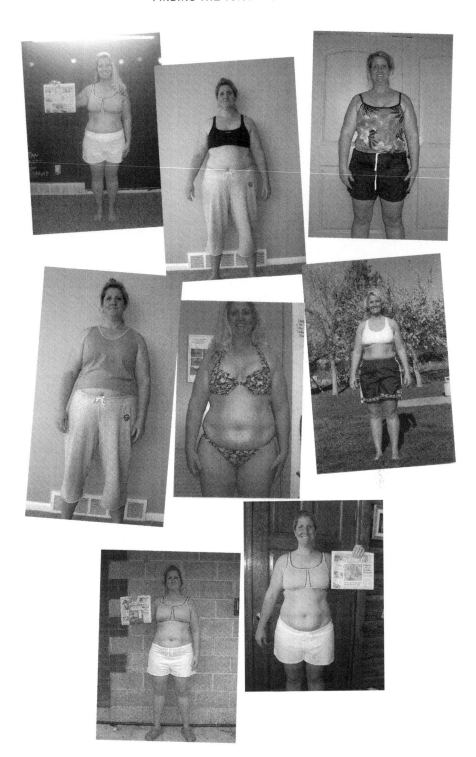

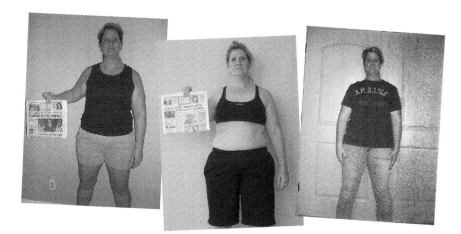

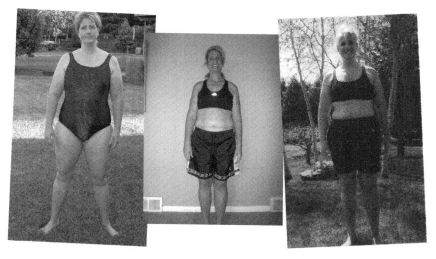

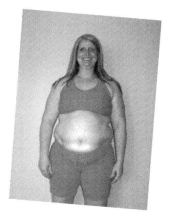
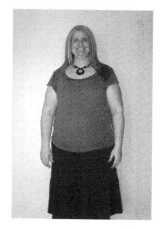

THE FIRST OF MANY AFTER PICTURES

Go confidently in the direction of your dreams!
Live the life you've imagined.

— Henry David Thoreau

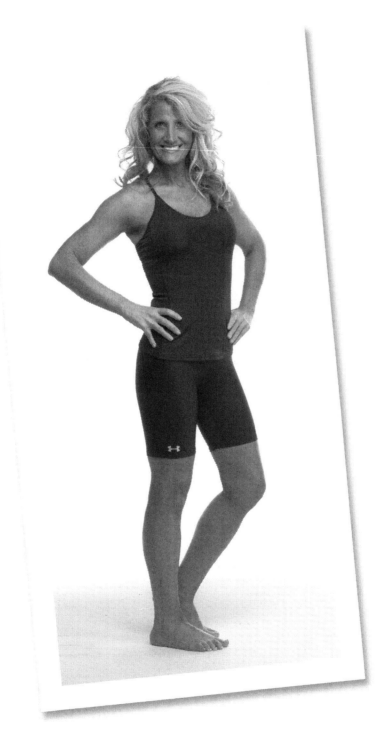

All our dreams can come true,
if we have the courage to pursue them.

— Walt Disney

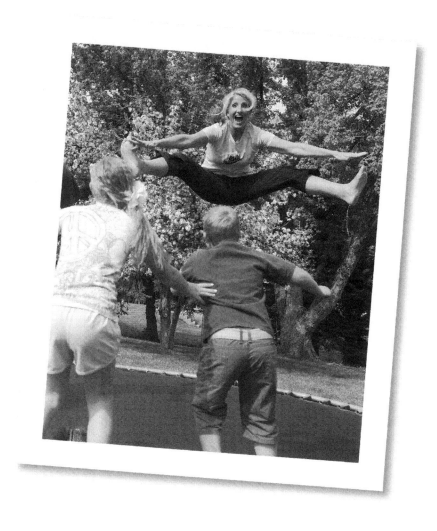

Have the courage to BE the person
you have always wanted to be,
the person God intends for you TO be.

— Jill Birth

16492394R10096

Made in the USA
Charleston, SC
23 December 2012